AF335465

AMERICAN MEDICINE IN CRISIS

Its Language and Philosophy

AMERICAN MEDICINE IN CRISIS

EDWARD P. LUONGO, M.D.

PHILOSOPHICAL LIBRARY
New York

Printed in the United States of America

DEDICATION

To those who helped and encouraged me most in this writing —my wife, Virginia Palmer Luongo, and my daughter, Mary Mather Dorsey.

CONTENTS

INTRODUCTION

In the art of healing, technical and social changes are occurring on a scale larger today than in its previous history. Need for reexamination of language exchanged among physicians and other members of society becomes apparent in light of some existing semantic impediments to general understanding of the dialogue.* In context even use of words "medical *care*" has different meaning for different people.

Meaning or, more properly, present impact of language and concepts employed by medicine require examination within present context and in relationship to medicine's history and philosophy. It has been through changes occurring in associative context and not logic that language in medicine derives its present meaning. Generally a large part of meaning in all language comes from continual changes in people, their social circumstances; cultures; the places and events involved.

Aristotle and Hippocrates affected the language and philosophy of medicine for many centuries with ethics, definitions, logic, and with wide spectrums of observations in natural, physical, and social sciences. Permeation of a variety of disciplines with Aristotelian logic caused much of human knowledge and language to become locked for over two thousand years in the lexicon of logic. Ancient and old-world doctrines, propositions, and concepts including those of Hippocrates became fossilized in "Permian" formations (the hidden "world" of events) while their usage survived

*Health always has been a hotly debated issue in America and a certain number of factors have combined at this time to make it an even greater source of controversy. The American "health" services are a good example of what can happen when such a vital topic is caught up in an ideologic straitjacket which one finds at the base of the "American Philosophy of Life."

with too few reexaminations of applicability to the new verbal world.

The writing of this book is no "search for sanity through language" (Korzsybski) in the physician-patient relationship*; nor is the book a *principia ethica* for practice of the healing art. There may never be a true "sanity" in a relationship in which both the healer and the patient "relate" to disease as human beings—albeit usually in different roles. There probably never can be a lasting, valid, all-encompassing *principia ethica* for practice of the healing art because of its cocultural evolution. The author shuns the role of innovator or reformer of professional actions, ethical systems, and protocols. He does believe a review of medicine's language, education, philosophy, and ethics in relation to present-day dialogues on health and medical care appears necessary.

Anthropologists find diverse arrays of ethical and social systems in different societies, which attest to the dynamics of evolution worked out in social structures "invented" by man. The old organic evolution, however, is not over; and though man may have attained his greatest increment in his cerebral size and weight when he reached the Neanderthal state, his brain pathway organization and complexity of higher neural functions continue to evolve.** In the meantime man's continued search for social and ethical canons continues to be geared to his evolution and to new designs of social structures.

The healing art conventionally could influence the direction of social evolution. In contributing to the direction of evolution in the social order, medical practitioners are handicapped at times by education, philosophy, and language. Their language does not always serve man's social aims in growth of interpersonal altruism. Since structures and content of language become reflected in behavior, physicians who speak in the arcane fashion of alchemists may

*Korzsybski hoped for revision of all sciences, particularly the sciences of man, in light of the non-Aristotelian notions he advocated. (Personal communication to author from J. Samuel Bois, May 1969.)

**These have been described in patterns resembling intricate reflexive pathways similar to those found by Pavlov in conditioning experiments with dogs.

behave in an obscure fashion. If they speak like economists they may behave according to the mores of the marketplace.

In the modern dialogue semantic ideation and orientation in language, philosophy, and education could improve teaching and practice of the healing art through better understanding of its verbal and nonverbal language. To explore some of the relationships between language, thought, and behavior in the healing art we first must consider those principles of its present-day language as they relate to the "territory" of experience of medicine as it has evolved to its present state.

In its evolution medicine and its language did not escape entirely some of the obfuscation created by the long conversation in progress among philosophers from the time of Aristotle to the present. Present-day medicine with its remnants of conservatism is now confronted with a philosophical dialogue in which "opposing forces" consider philosophy and language as a means of not only *understanding* but actively *changing* the world.

The inexact science and the art of medicine have brought untold benefits to human beings as individuals yet its "organizations" find it a difficult task to "sell" medical practice as a segment of free enterprise.* Medicine's immense accomplishment in healing the sick has been exceeded only by its willing but inadequate social commitment.** Some of the inadequacy stems from a nostalgic image of its traditions and language. It has been unable to forget its past even amidst the battle going on within its ranks between stereotypes (thesis) of the past and forces of antithesis. Whether the healing art can abandon its nostalgia, modify its self-concept, will be tested by those who challenge both political and social

*A new battle is shaping up with lines drawn between the opposing forces of organized medicine and government; this could prove longer and more bitter than previous encounters in the political arena.

**Of late (December 1969) organized medicine has been pressured by social forces to provide leadership in the nation's effort to improve the quantity and quality of health services rendered to the poor. Basic to the plan are the concepts of citizens' rights to adequate medical care and rights to choose physicians and institutions in the delivery of medical care.

tenets in our society. In any event, it may be a sad climb to the attic when medicine must sift through its heirlooms, both useful and useless, of philosophy, educational systems, and language, deciding which to save and which to discard.*

Much in this book is not new, but like most writing, a synthesis of what has been said about words, ideas, and people by many other writers many times. Part of the book is devoted to how medicine's heirlooms became lodged in the attic; more of it deals with the sorting through. To do this we must consider first medicine's evolutionary process beginning with traditions of the ancient world up to its modern practice. Closely allied are changes occurring in self-concept and philosophy of the practitioner—also his research, inventions, his utterances, and his attitudes conscious or unconscious in relationship to social and cultural change. We will consider the healing art's resistance to new ideas and social change in light of some nondynamic characteristics in its philosophy and education. Associated with this resistance are problems in medicine's intra- and extramural communications especially in the field of psychiatry and in the delivery of medical care. Finally we will consider the paths ahead for the healing art in the new psychosocial disorder prevalent in society.

*Already, leadership in organized medicine is beginning to speak of altering "cherished" traditions and practices of its membership so as to accept and support totally new ideas whether these be devised by physicians or those outside the profession.

INTRODUCTION

American Medical Assoc. News. Weekly editions (1966-1969).

Bois, J. Samuel. *Explorations in Awareness.* New York, Evanston, and London: Harper & Row, 1957.

Bryson, Lyman, *et al.* (eds.). *Symbols and Society.* New York: Harper & Brothers, 1955.

Chapin, Miriam. *How People Talk.* New York: The John Day Company, 1945.

Cohen, Robert. "Language and Behaviour." *American Scientist,* vol. 49 (1961).

de Chardin, Teilhard. *The Phenomenon of Man.* New York and Evanston: Harper & Row, 1961.

Hayakawa, S. I. *Language in Thought and Action.* New York: Harcourt, Brace, 1949.

Hayakawa, S. I. (ed.). *The Use and Misuse of Language.* Greenwich: Fawcett Publications, Inc., 1962.

Korzybski, Alfred. *Science and Sanity: An Introduction to Non-Aristotelian Systems and General Semantics,* 3rd ed. International Non-Aristotelian Library Publishing Co., 1948.

Language, Thought and Reality: Selected Writings of B. L. Whorf, ed. John B. Carroll. New York: Wiley, 1956.

Lee, Irving. *Language Habits in Human Affairs.* New York: Harper & Brothers, 1941.

Magoun, H. W., Darling, Louise; Prost, J. The Evolution of Man's Brain. New York: Josiah Macy Jr. Foundation, 1960.

Wild, John. *The Challenge of Existentialism.* Bloomington: Indiana University Press, 1951.

Wilson, Richard A. *The Miraculous Birth of Language.* New York: Philosophical Library, 1948.

What's wrong with U. S. medicine, The plight of the U. S. patient. *Time* 93:53-58, 1969.

CHAPTER I

The Ancient and Modern Worlds of Medicine —

Their Evolution in Social, Philosophic, and Technologic Contexts

When modern medicine looks to past traditions and their custody, it sees a heritage, historically, mostly glorious but sometimes inglorious, noble and at times ignoble. Its traditions have different meaning for different persons, depending upon vantage points or from which contexts medicine's evolution is viewed.

Medicine's modern intra- and extramural dialogue retains coloration of ancient heritages. Some traditions have become obsolete in relation to the present-day practice of the healing art; though having validity within original historical context, some old traditions lack meaning when applied to modern problems; i.e., in delivery of medical care, ethics, and philosophy and its educational systems. Medicine's history must be reckoned with, however, to understand its cocultural or cosocial evolution and its language. Reckoning with the ancient and modern worlds of medicine sheds light on some of medicine's present-day semantic difficulties having origin in its history, philosophy, and system of education.

Ancient documents (the Edwin Smith and Eber Papyruses) give little insight as to scope or limitations placed upon medicine and surgery by the pharaohs.* Imhotep trephined (bored holes in) human skulls on the banks of the Nile sixty centuries ago; this surgery was as much a religious exercise as one of healing. So great was the religious implication, Imhotep was worshipped as a god by Egyptians for centuries after his death. Whether he performed surgery for simple headaches or brain tumors, Imhotep's godliness was proclaimed especially by patients who survived. Perhaps historically this represents the instance when medicine and surgery first became unfairly burdened with the warranty of deity.

The Smith and Eber Papyruses reveal, in the practice of Egyptian medicine, the concept of hygiene, emphasizing cleanliness of persons, dwellings, and cities and regulated by law. Hygienic measures such as furnishing animal-bladder respirators to stone cutters working in pyramid dust may have been less a tribute to the pharaoh's benevolence or morality than to a sense of urgency and expediency and his interest in a monument to himself.

Parallel civilizations in Mesopotamia, Babylon, and Assyria offered "benefits" of the healing art copied from Egyptian medicine and surgery. Little detail is known of medicine or surgery performed in these countries. Surgery was considered a craft, and very little craft lore is contained in cuneiform writings. The earliest references to medical economics and jurisprudence is found in Hammurabi's code of law (1800 B.C.). The code prescribed fees for surgeons in amounts of two to 10 shekels as compared to a mechanic's annual wage of eight shekels and stipulated penalties to surgeons for unsuccessful operations (even removal of the surgeon's hand).

*It was not until the beginning of the thirteenth century that scope and skill in medical practice became regulated through examination procedures. These procedures were decreed by royal edict at the Collegium Salensis [Salerno] Medical School, in order that patients not incur the "hazards" due to lack of skill of physicians. Examinations were not written but were of the conversational type between student and teachers; this test of skill was given for over five hundred years in Europe. Not until the eighteenth century were written examinations required to test the skill and judgment of students and practitioners of the healing art. Even in modern times there existed, until very recently, regulations such as those found in Mexico, which required that aspiring practitioners need only publicly advertise their *lack* of diploma or license in order to practice the healing art.

Greek medicine in its modalities transcended advances of previous civilizations. That Greeks like the Egyptians made gods of their "physicians" is of semantic significance. An early semantic disaster for medicine occurred when the "serpent" and "staff" were placed in the hands of a Thessalian chieftain Asklepios, making him the god of medicine. The Aescalapean staff (caduceus) with its snake symbolism was to become a symbol of dread and awe among the Greek and later civilizations.

The earliest evidences of class distinction in quality of medical care are found in Plato's *Republic*. Slaves, because of station in life, were less worthy of medical care than free citizens. Plato gives to the physician an earthly, "authoritarian" symbolism requiring that "the sick man, be he rich or poor, attend at the physician's door" just as all who require governing must "attend at the gate of him who is able to govern."

Under a plane tree on Cos Hippocrates practiced medicine among large numbers of people, many of whom traveled great distances to attend at his door. The "mound of communication," the Hippocratic plane tree, was accessible to the multitudes and access to the healer was "horizontal."* Hippocrates was not hampered by "vertical"** Minoan labyrinths encountered in modern medical communications. During this period of his medical practice Hippocrates furnished medicine ethical canons, its oath, and a basis for its philosophy. He admonished other physicians "not to be anxious about fixing a fee and not seek a profit but lay hold a reputation."*** He reminded them "where there is love of

---

*Head to head and feet to feet contacts of people.

**Head to feet contacts found in vertical structures. See Doxiadis, C. A., "Man and the Space Around Him," *Saturday Review,* (Dec. 14) 1968.

***"Sometimes give your services for nothing, calling to mind a previous benefaction or present satisfaction. And if there be an opportunity of serving one who is a stranger in financial straits, give full assistance to all such. For where there is love of man, there is also love of the art. For some patients, though conscious that their condition is perilous, recover their health simply through their contentment with the goodness of the physician. And it is well to superintend the sick to make them well, to care for one's self, so as to observe what is seemly."—Hippocrates, *Precepts,* Chap. 6.

man there is also love of the art" and that they should serve strangers in financial straits.

Hippocrates propounded a hygiene based on the "morality" and ethics of hedonism; hygiene was based on the premise that "he who lives well is blessed and happy, and that he who lives otherwise is the reverse." Whether the "owner of happiness" was happy or unhappy often was lost in sophistry. Greek philosophers considered gymnastic training, *submission* to medical treatment in illness, as well as the practice of medicine irksome yet beneficial. It is difficult to conclude from Greek philosophical discussions who benefited more—the healer or the seeker of healing.

Hippocrates discoursed on ethical* and technical criteria applicable to the medical care of all classes. Medicine as practiced by Hippocrates, however, was limited in application mainly to the leisured class. His thesis *Airs, Waters, Places* for example has great significance in the history of environmental health. Nevertheless this was written not for the "dishonored, socially stigmatized" working classes but for aristocrats enjoying the privileges of Greek liberty. By careful study Hippocrates sought a balance between his patients and their environments. He regarded illness as a disturbance in the equilibrium of nature in which the physician must "cooperate" with nature to reestablish proper balance between patients' internal and external environments. This was sought frequently in the prescription of food intake and exercise.

---

*"I swear by Apollo the Physician, by Aesculapius, by Health, by Panacea, and by all the gods and goddesses, making them my witnesses, that I will carry out, according to my ability and judgment, this oath and this indenture. To hold my teacher in this art equal to my own parents; to make him partner in my livelihood; when he is in need of money to share mine with him; to consider his family as my own brothers, and to teach them this art, if they want to learn it, without fee or indenture. I will use treatment to help the sick according to my ability and judgment, but never with a view to injury and wrongdoing. I will keep pure and holy both my life and my art. In whatsoever houses I enter, I will enter to help the sick, and I will abstain from all intentional wrongdoing and harm. And whatsoever I shall see or hear in the course of my profession in my intercourse with men, if it be what should not be published abroad, I will never divulge, holding such things to be holy secrets. Now if I carry out this oath, and break it not, may I gain forever reputation among all men for my life and for my art; but if I transgress it and forswear myself, may the opposite befall me."—Hippocrates, trans. by William Henry Rich Jones (1817-1885).

The diets (pork, mutton, lamb, pheasant) suggested by Hippocrates hardly if ever were in reach of the slave, potter, or peasant; the exercise (long walks three times daily) had little relevance to slaves who walked all day.

Much semantic awareness in Greek medicine and culture is constricted by writings of philosophers and physician-philosophers of the age with "peculiar" social opportunities and attitudes derived from their observation of events and public affairs. Plato had every advantage of training, being the son of rich parents, robust in health, and educated in all the accomplishments of the time. While fully versed in the philosophy of the nature of justice and injustice, the need for labor and its division in society, his awareness was colored by his liberty and freedom as a Greek citizen. This citizenship for centuries disfranchised workers, most of whom were slaves. Socrates looked upon them as bad friends and patriots, degenerated physically and spiritually by labor; socially stigmatized; and rightly dishonored in Greek cities. These were the class limitations of Hippocratic medicine; i.e., the favoring of citizen physicians with citizen patients to the exclusion of the working man. Thus medicine in its early origins lacked total social commitment, and this was expressed in its early language.

The Hippocratic system of medicine was adopted by Roman and successive civilizations. Galen, the last of the ancient Greek physicians, was to carry on the Greek tradition in Rome. He remained an idol, his writings *sacrosanct*, through the darkness of the Middle Ages until the "discoverer" of human anatomy, Vesalius, "tore the Galen idol down."

Many causes have been attributed to the fall of the Roman Empire, including the boredom of an indolent citizenry, lacking challenge, and lead poisoning among successive generations of politicians drinking wine from metal utensils. The despair of its citizenry made many in the empire receptive to the ideology and philosophy of Christianity. Mythological figures both Greek and Roman were replaced. The priests and priestesses of the Aesculaepial cult were forgotten. The practice of healing became identified with Christian evangelism in Europe, North Africa, and Asia Minor. We find healing practiced as a combined profession of

Christian priesthood and medicine. "Scientific" medicine remained centuries away and experimental inquiry into the nature of disease was regarded as a culpable activity.* The Christian, unlike the early Graeco and Roman tradition, in medicine embraced free citizens and slaves alike.

Medicine remained within a religious context during the Middle Ages. Like other intellectual disciplines it was subject to the censorship of Christian dogmas, which limited spread of knowledge to what would contribute to man's salvation. The dominance of dogma gave man's earthly existence a vertical component toward the heavens; his horizontal component (earthliness) was considered secondary, and relatively unimportant.

The context of medicine became intimately bound to an aura of miracles, divine revelation, and sainthood—an aura, partially remaining in the legacy of medicine today. Two physicians, Cosmas and Damian, were venerated as saints for miraculous cures of sickness in men and animals. They died as martyrs in 287 A.D. during the reign of Diocletian. The Christian world since has accepted them as patrons (saints) of physicians, surgeons, and pharmacists. It is notable that the first interracial organ transplant was attributed to Saints Cosmas and Damian in a Roman legend, which depicts a leg transplant from a deceased black Moor to a white devout Christian. The Christian had lost a leg from "cancer," a term used in the early Christian era for any condition that destroyed skin and flesh.**

In his *Historia Naturalis*, a classical encyclopedia of natural science, Pliny the Elder (23-70 A.D.) furnishes very little insight into condition of the healing art in Rome except his mention of inhalation and comments on breech presentations in obstetrics. During the years of the dark ages or gloomy fog (caeca nebula), described by Vergil, the halls of medicine were illumined only by

*Here the thought control (exercised in the name of salvation) at times far exceeded the rigorousness of any seen in modern dictatorships of Nazi, Marxist, or communistic countries.

**The eighteenth century physician, Hermann Boerhaave, gives in his book, *Aphorisms,* the scientific description of cancer as "having the likeness to a crab."

the flickering tapers of Galen's writings. This second century Greek physician who practiced in Rome was influenced not by Christianity but by Judaic monotheism. He combined Judaism with Hippocratic principles and Aristotelian philosophy. His teleologic dogmatism depicting the purpose of the body exclusively as an instrument of the soul won virtually canonical support of the Christian church.

Practice of the healing art became a skill in the "sophistry of taboo" in which the writings of Galen and church dogma were pitted against any new concepts (technical or social) that might arise. This state of affairs in medicine was to persist until the Copernican thought "revolution," which later led to the seventeenth-century rebirth of medicine and natural science. The semantic imprint of Galen on the healing art lingers today in reactionism of thought and language; at times in extreme distrust of social or technical innovation.

Rising from a culture with no indigenous philosophy and at times ruthless and cruel as the land's barren deserts, Arabian medicine took hold in Asia Minor, North Africa, and parts of Europe invaded by the Moslems. Though its general philosophy and medicine were borrowed from the Greeks, Syrians, and Iberians, Arabic medicine developed in an atmosphere far more free than that of salvation-conscious European medievalism. Greek works on medicine were improved upon translation and shorn of much of their deism and classicism. Arabic writing explored greater areas of awareness through its close association with general philosophy. The Persian Ibn Sina (980-1037 A.D., known to the western world as Avicenna), though at times debauched and by no means a saintly character, was the greatest physician of the time. He was a product of this resurgence of medicine among the Arabs and taught both medicine and philosophy at Teheran and Ispahan.

The adventuresome philosophical explorations of Arab physicians, recognizing no bounds in either sophistic taboos, Christian dogma, or Aristotelian Galenism, stimulated progressive attitudes later among European Renaissance physicians with regard to learning generally and medicine particularly. Of note also in the resurgence of medicine in Arab countries were two Cordoban physician-philosophers, Moses Mamonides (Moisés de Mamon, 1135-1204 A.D.) and Averroës (1126-1196), both of whom were "imported" as medical advisers to Moslem potentates. Averroës had introduced Aristotelian thought to the west and later was identified with the Arabic system of medicine. Moses Mamonides, as brilliant an intellectual as Iberia has produced, combined philosophy with medicine in his writings, whose subjects ranged from asthma to the "hygiene of living in a healthful manner without medicine" to the principles of sexual intercourse.

Later Arabic medicine was to experience restraint of religious dogma when the caliph Yaqub Al-Mansur became alarmed at the unorthodoxy of Arabic medicine, especially that of Averroës. He was exiled on the basis that "God had decreed hellfire for those who thought truth could be found by unaided reason"; all books on logic and metaphysics were burned.

During the early Renaissance and through the seventeenth century Galen idols were toppled one by one by the prime alchemist, Paracelsus,* and later by Vesalius and Malpighi, the anatomists; Harvey, "discoverer" of blood circulation; and Ramazzini, the environmentalist.

Most notable of the late or post-Renaissance physicians was Ramazzini whose awareness of social conditions of his times did much to harmonize the language and tendencies of medicine with the social order. He was first among physicians in effecting a cocentricity of medicine to the social order. His concern was for man's total environment in relationship to illness. This was to prove to be a most glorious and revolutionary innovation, which furnished medicine a lasting ideology two thousand years after Hippocrates.

In his *De Morbus Artifius Diatriba (Diseases of Occupations)* Ramazzini admonished practitioners of the healing art to expand their constricted Hippocratic awareness of patients, rich and poor, by showing interest in total living situations in the community,

*Aureolus Philippus Theophrastus Bombastus von Hohenheim, a leader of the Rosicrucian movement in Austria.

particularly man at work. Ramazzini visited patients both at home and at work. He knew well health hazards facing the cesspit workers of his native city, Modena, since he observed them directly at work and later cared for them at home.

While respecting hygiene standards of the city of Modena he knew that cost of the workmen who spent four hours a day in this type of work—"It was as bad as going blind." While convinced of the importance to the progress of civilization of the mechanical arts Ramazzini was impressed by the wretched working conditions endured by those involved. These "arts" caused grave injury to the artisan, who by seeking to support life and raise a family, often received from his work a fatal disease and died cursing his craft.

In his attempts to harmonize language and tendencies of the healing art with problems of the social order Ramazzini was convinced that medicine had an obligation (shared by jurisprudence) to contribute to the solution of social problems. He admonished his colleagues to work toward reforms affecting the psychosocial order when conditions in the order are detrimental to the well-being of its members. Thus Ramazzini initiated the overthrow in the art of healing of many class limitations imposed by Hippocratic medicine. Succeeding generations of practitioners were to deal with the environments of the commoner and aristocrat alike and gain knowledge of entire disease groups affecting those living under unhealthful conditions in cities and those working in factories and mines.

In the eighteenth century Edward Jenner, a physician with interests ranging from geology to ornithology, followed the Ramazzinian precept in accurate observation of the total environment of patients. His masterly powers of observation led to the discovery of occupationally-induced cowpox immunity among milkmaids and the development of smallpox vaccine.

From 1746, in England and other countries, the healing art found new commitment and language in the social and economic ferment of industrialization and among a rapidly swelling lower middle class of factory workers. The stage was set for important observations relating to occupational disease, puerperal or child-bed-fever, tuberculosis, typhus, and other diseases in relationship to population groups.

The early nineteenth century physician, Charles Turner Thackrah, by close association with the humanitarian, Robert Owen, became interested in medical problems and social evils resulting from the mode of production in the new industrialism of the times. Thackrah was largely responsible for inculcating among his medical colleagues, the public, and government a sense of moral responsibility and social commitment toward reform, with regard to prevention of diseases and social evils. When he established a new School of Medicine at Leeds he opposed the monopoly in medical education (curative medicine) held by the two royal colleges in London. Thackrah brought to the new medical educational system at Leeds his personal philosophy and a language of social commitment: "Each master . . . has in great measure the health and happiness of his workpeople in his power . . . let benevolence be directed to the prevention, rather than to the relief, of the evils [sickness and social degradation] which our civic state so widely and deeply produces." Semantically the language of the modern American public health movement traces much of its import to Thackrah's preoccupation with inciting social reforms as they related to both prevention and cure of disease and social ills.*

The nineteenth century discoveries of Pasteur, Koch, and their practical applications by Lister gave new meaning to "public health," which during the twentieth century was to change much of medicine. The public health concept accrued semantic importance for it originated from observations of health problems among large population groups. Pasteur, Koch, and Virchow produced within the context of the healing art an awareness of "unit" causes and relationships of microorganisms to disease and diseased tissues to symptoms in illness. The application of unit concepts in disease revolutionized medicine and surgery. These

*In American medicine, in the early and middle twentieth century, we find a notable counterpart to Dr. Thackrah in the person of Dr. Alice Hamilton who brought about significant reforms related to the social ills and health hazards of factory workers.

advancements were not without shortcomings; their nonholistic conceptual by-products were to plague the healing art to the present day. Employing Aristotelian logic reinforced by Newtonian philosophy (units of action and his scientific method) the total human body became the sum of its parts.

Various discliplines were given scientific meaning by "mechanic" unit explanations by fragmentation of their totality.* Thus the working atoms of chemistry became dynamic units explaining subject and substance. The "atoms" of biology were first considered to be cells, chromosomes, genes, nucleic acids, and later helical arrangements of purine pyrimidine bases with attached sugar phosphate radicals. In psychology and neurology the simplest dynamic unit forces were considered instincts, synapses, primary reflexes; and later in psychiatry units were sought by postulation in an egg-shaped model of the ego, super ego, the id.** This fragmentation affected political science and economics.

So too in medicine; the human body became subject to mechanical unit explanation (tissue, cells, endocrine secretions, proteins, sugars, minerals, macromolecules and molecules). In man consideration of unit function "mechanisms" superseded consideration of these functions in relationship to total function and "purpose." Mechanistic explanation cannot fully clarify the "cooperative" synchronization of these units in preservation of the purpose of the whole human organism within its environment. Though logic dictated that study of the "pieces" would lead to understanding of total organism economy, this became questionable in the same sense as the "understanding" of Greek temples through study of marble blocks. Only as one views the totality of molecules as structurally and functionally synchronized in walls and columns of the body does the human structure and sanctuary take on holistic

---

*See Harry Prosch, *Genesis of Twentieth Century Philosophy, The Evolution of Thought from Copernicus to the Present.* Garden City: Doubleday and Co., Inc., 1964.

**In the feverish writing of his great "Project" (Theory of the Mind), Freud clung desperately, at first, to the concept that the mind could be described in terms of neurons and synapses and ultimately in the language of chemistry, physics, and mathematics. See Ernest Jones, *The Life and Work of Sigmund Freud.* New York: Basic Books, 1953.

form. If through discovery man becomes able to unlock secrets of the tiniest and humblest to the most magnificent "house" of life, many ultimate questions will remain unanswered, particularly ones in the realm of the "noble" workings of the human brain.

Specialization of interest or awareness in the isolated function of body parts and tissue conceptually has led medicine further from the total human structure as a sanctuary. Increased awareness of units and parts made physicians less philosophical in the direction of ultimate realities of life and living. In this manner the art of healing became an art and science of units and parts. It largely ignored philosophical skepticism and its reservations concerning "substance" (little atoms with empty spaces between them). Such explanations still lead us to ask, How much space in terms of electronic orbits do fear and anxiety occupy in the human body?

Those most responsible for the scientific revolution in medicine (through mechanistic and unit discovery) warned against dehumanization of the art through its fragmentation. Koch, by example in demographic exploration, and Virchow by dictum held that medicine was a social science. They emphasized throughout their lifetimes the necessity for the practitioner to have a "Weltanschauung" of the human being as a whole, including his social and biological purpose. In their own fatherland this admonition went largely unheeded.* Clinical medicine in Germany at the beginning of the twentieth century became dehumanized. Many clinical teachers were too engrossed in physiology, bacteriology, pathology, and biochemistry; they no longer looked at the patient or said "Good morning" when he came into the consulting room.

Today there exists within medicine's context of awareness "social medicine,"** applied by the British to "preventive" medicine and "public health." This deals with the study of distribution and

*In Germany (Wilhelm Fliess) and Austria, at the turn of the nineteenth century, many leading teachers and clinicians (especially the Breuer, Freud [early], Meynert and Brücke group) were strong adherents of the Helmholtz school, which strove to describe medicine ultimately in terms of physics and mathematics. See Ernest Jones, *The Life and Work of Sigmund Freud.* New York: Basic Books, 1953.

**Originally termed "political medicine" in the 1850's; later, in 1870, called "state medicine," and at turn of the century, "public health."

behavior of diseases in human populations; definition of agents responsible for disease patterns; and the modifying effects of social or environmental conditions on the evolution of disease patterns. In brief a new language evolved, concentric with sociology. There is also "socialized medicine," where semantic difficulties are greatest and where organized medicine, government, and social action forces in labor and public health are in dispute. Stripped of rhetoric, the progressive purposes of both social medicine and socialized medicine are to furnish the greatest amount of good to the greatest number of people. While tolerating *social medicine* the organized society of medicine continues to fight *socialized medicine*. Social medicine seemed less of a threat since it dealt with preventive modalities in which few physicians had interest—albeit in the past a large number of physicians considered these modalities a corrupting influence on the pure practice of curative medicine. The term socialized medicine, though semantically progressive, becomes more than controversial since it deals mainly with curative aspects of medical care, the prime interests of most physicians professionally and economically. Meanwhile the language of prevention and cure becomes progressively denuded of meaning in the evolution of the healing art. The fine line of demarcation between preventive and curative medicine has become blurred; medicine's language of social commitment (social or socialized), is complicated by a multitude of conflicting philosophies (economic and political) within its own ranks.

Those in academic circles of medicine hope to restore semantic sanity to the medical language by effecting a greater concentricity between medicine and the humanities, the behavioral and social sciences. Hoped for is a resurgence of holistic concepts that recognize disease causality in areas of deprivation other than organic or physiological among individual emotional, social, and other needs of human beings. Also hoped for is a more suitable language for future practitioners of the healing art. These hopes are threatened by antithetical forces of "specialism" and "generalism." Forces of specialism strengthened of late by "researchism" keep growing in number as survival of many medical teaching institutions continues to depend on funded research.

Funded research in teaching institutions brings with it an awareness and language cognitive of mathematics, computer technology, the physical sciences. Specialism and mechanistic medical philosophy continue to flourish among those engaged in long-term experimental observation of phenomena limited to small groups of cells, tissue molecules, or atoms.

Impressed by precise methodology of those limiting their interests to unit phenomena, many students and practitioners develop nonemotive language and awareness of the healing art, which channels them toward specialization. Potentiating channelization is the symbolic language of computers, electron microscopes, and an array of scientific instruments ranging from hemodialysers to cardiac monitoring systems. Interest in seeking knowledge of the "questionable" becomes supplanted by pursuit of the unequivocal." The seeking of unequivocal "facts of medicine" through purely technological frames of reference may discourage constructive speculation. This in turn impairs integrative skill and correlation of realities met in clinical presence. Often, what is seen is not the nature of the total human being but that part exposed to the particular technique of observation. Thus much of the profession, in overreacting or overcompensating to a long history of empiricism of the pre-Osler era, employs methods and language of science to an inordinate degree, in a profession considered to be both art and an inexact science.

The modern-day healing art is faced with patients having scientific expectations yet who continue to ask wistfully, "whatever became of the old-fashioned doctor." The logic of the dilemma suggests that something old and inferior has been supplanted by something new and superior. However, the nonlogical structure of language and emotions may convey the feeling that something new and inferior has been added to the healing art.

The practice of the healing art, in its present stage of evolution, consists of both "new-fashioned" physicians and patients. Its dilemma lies in the ambivalent expectations of the modern patient who believes strongly in medical progress through science and specialism yet rejects those dehumanizing or impersonal aspects of modern practice. Some patients feel they must make a flat choice between an understanding or more "qualified" doctor. Within this aura of patient thought and language it becomes futile to maintain that "logic dictates" a choice between impersonal technical proficiency and more humanistic but less proficient physician care.

It would seem that humanistic understanding of both the generalist (for personal and psychological guidance) and the more detached, though often better qualified, specialist are necessary. Educational means could supply this except that the imbalance in interest among students weighs heavily in favor of science and specialism while the opportunity to serve the holistic concept of man generally proves unattractive. Specialism practiced in the vertical communication mounds of large medical centers also proves more attractive to students than the horizontal mounds of neighborhood practice.

With threat of dehumanization and a declining ratio of physicians interested in dealing with the sociocultural behavior of patients, we find the healing art in a precarious situation. This comes at a time when dehumanizing political and social forces are prevalent in society. Those practitioners who assert, as some do, they "have no use for emotion" under present conditions in society in effect abdicate the human race. They become part of a growing number of human beings who ignore the conspectus of a million years in human history, both physical and cultural—a conspectus of how man came to be as he is now.

The future of *humanitas* in medicine depends on new generations of physicians who choose commitment to living a life of love for the cause of mankind whether they do this simply out of love for all or in a religious sense for the love of God. Meanwhile in the present-day language of science versus humanity we note phrases and questions such as: Can the art of medicine survive; The case for theoretical medicine; Sciences of new importance to medicine; Expanding dimensions in medicine; The patient in medical education; Anthropology in medical education; Whatever became of the old-fashioned patient; Whatever became of the old-fashioned doctor; Training for family medicine; Computer medicine; Computer diagnosis; The telephone company's case for long-distance diagnosis; We can't attract young graduates into family practice because they have had no exposure to good family practitioners; Physicians back plans to upgrade care; Negro physicians form own group; Physicians! Speak as one voice; A challenge exists, but no blueprint; Involve the public; Stand up and be counted; What are the moral, religious, and legal aspects of organ transplantations; Is Hippocrates really relevant to modern medicine; Should physicians go on strike; Has modern medicine reversed Hippocratic procedures; Do practitioners of the healing art really "practice" on patients; and, Is the reversal of the Hippocratic role due to the economics of fees for service.

One solution for the science versus humanity dilemma in medicine would structure its educational system according to special spheres of awareness: research, specialism, and teaching, and general or family practice. This would be accomplished in undergraduate and graduate training curricula. Symbolism of arrangement suitable for research activity, specialization, and teacher training would be lodged in the large vertical communication mounds of modern medical centers. This, however, would be unsuitable for training of generalists. Brought into these vertical mounds to teach, generalists become sorely hampered in teaching family medicine away from a normal community setting. Only to the extent that medical centers could provide satellite models of community milieus is there any hope for effective teaching of family medicine. Conceivably two genera of institutions may be necessary: one teaching the art of medicine in a rural locale; the other teaching the science of medicine in an urban locale, with urban and rural suburban patients doing without one or the other.

Another dilemma in modern healing lies in the relationship of the practitioner to "nature." Is the modern practitioner's role an auxiliary one to nature? If so, has modern medicine become too activist in character? Much of Hippocrates' therapeutic relevance lay in his reverence for nature as a prime healer. He used the word "nature" semantically as the subject of either a transitive or intransitive verb. This made the physician "para" to nature, a relationship given conscious or unconscious acceptance historically in the tradition of the healing art. Physicians willingly or not "cooperated" with the forces of nature in their therapeutic regimens.

With modern advances in surgical techniques, medical biology, immunology, antibiotics, and drug therapy, physicians have become more and more antagonists of nature.* They actively combat natural forces that tend to effect a homeostasis of the human organism within its internal and external environments. Some unrecognized forces are extinctional; their displacement (as in immusuppression used in organ transplants) causes body protests in the form of substituted symptom disease complexes (S.S.D.C.) and rejection of the "good" for the "bad." The question here is whether or not the activist physician is doing something good for nature; i.e., something nature would like to do for herself, if she could.

Knowledge of what nature wants *in any particular* organism may be locked in individual genetic programming among the human species. "Nature" may be possessed of true neuroticism in that certain stimuli of the past may become defeating, even death-dealing forces of the present or future in the organism's responsiveness. Modern medicine frequently faces the task of changing nature's mind and genetic codes and combatting or thwarting its destructive responses, sometimes by none-too-gentle means. Those means temporarily hide nature's intentions and what nature would like may be temporarily or permanently lost to view. Involved are nature's internal radial (directional within) tendencies in the human organism, tendencies harbored in genetic codes that may forebode future evolution of "the could" in man.

Since nature to a degree has been identified with both "good" and "bad" forces acting within man's internal and external environments, we can no longer insist on the traditional role of the physician (phusis-) as para- or ancillary to nature. The evolution of his role has become more and more, through technical advancement, one of antagonist rather than protagonist of nature's work; at times this makes boobery of "body wisdom."

---

*This is especially true in the use of drugs given to well persons to prevent "something"; i.e., birth control pills, anticholesterol drugs and preventive vaccines, all of which at times have undesirable effects on the well person.

It would be unthinkable however to cast man in general and the physician particularly in a role of a detached, inactive bystander witnessing effects of natural forces acting upon him. In countering natural forces, man learned to use shelter, fire, and antiseptics. He is too taken up by power of invention to be a passive witness to natural forces. The modern physician through invention has learned to monitor and control these forces and in doing so becomes less a handmaiden of nature and more a prime healer. He hopes by careful monitoring to forestall the disaster of natural and directional forces in the human organism at times when nature may "wish" renewal of species and death of the organism. As a monitor, the physician with the patient and all those associated with him become caught up in sophisticated systems of dials, clocks, and readings.

In modern patient care settings where complex technology, cybernetics, and automation are introduced in monitoring, the "world of events" of the patient (personal interactions with other human beings) may seem of less concern than the quality, precision, and continuity in his evaluation. To patients not prepared for this experience psychologically, wires, tubes, catheters, and electrodes symbolically can speak a frightening language of scientific, precise, but impersonal medical care. Thus the early dictum of careful and *personal* observation pronounced by Hippocrates and in more modern times by Florence Nightingale remains a basic humanistic principle in modern patient *care*, even though monitoring of patients has become more precise and automatic.

In considering the physician in his modern role as the prime healer in relation to nature we must look also at activism in modern medical practice. To "do something, whatever it is" is the demand of our activist culture, and this infusion of activism at times reverses Hippocratic criteria in medicine. The leading role as activists naturally would go to surgical specialists. The "handworking" of the surgeon (*cheirergon* or *chirurgia*) has remained through the ages a highly regarded mechanical skill. Skill required in recommending nonintervention in a particular disease often proves less highly regarded in activist cultures. Also held in lesser regard is skill in pondering sociocultural behavior of patients, which because of its intangibility to them often becomes less worthy of a fee.

Surgical skill in its most integrative sense involves judgment and skill within the triad of pathology, procedure, and general health of the patient, in relation to morbidity and mortality statistics. In addition surgery is an instrument of final diagnosis. We have also, in a different sense, the skill of gauging calculated risk related to "presumptive" diagnosis, as when surgeons at one time proceeded to remove a normal appendix to avoid risk of rupture of an abnormal one. Surgical removal of normal tissue at times was termed truly lifesaving in that it overcame the calculated risk of rupture. While to some this was bad medicine, to many good surgeons it was good surgery.

Much of the militant activism in the history of American medicine was connected with the signing of the Declaration of Independence. Dr. Benjamin Rush (1745-1813), one of the signers, captured the spirit of 1776 both in a patriotic and professional sense. Like Ambroise Paré (1517-'90), the surgeon serving French kings on the battlefield, Dr. Rush's awareness was colored by the perpetual state of exhilaration and exaltation he experienced during the stirring scenes of the times. He taught thousands of students and gave direction to the evolution of American medicine, infusing his followers with a sense of impatience with nature and *aequinimitas* and the desire to conduct "heroic" practices. He caught the value systems of the times steeped in sanguine enterprise, confidence, audacity, bowie knives, revolvers, and Fourth-of-July orations. The social order in America and elsewhere has not evolved sufficiently, even today, to develop socioeconomic and ethical safeguards for heroic practice in the healing art.

The exhilaration felt by Dr. Rush is matched today by surgical pioneers who have captured the spirit of those beginning to penetrate space, in their advancement of surgical techniques in organ transplantation. The consequences to the social order will not be known until the techniques are proven permanently useful to man.* From the time of Doctors Rush, McDowell, and Agnew to

*Even if these techniques are perfected, medically and surgically, only a small percentage (16%) of the estimated 200,000 Americans, under the

the more modern surgeons Halstead, Babcock, Mayo, DeBakey, Barnard and Cooley the healing art has been and is caught up in the technical awareness of the times well in advance of full exploration of socioeconomic implications. Modern technical excellence has produced not only living organ transplants but mechanical devices capable of taking over faltering functions of diseased organs. Patients "chosen" to receive the benefits of such devices are few compared to the number needing them. The limited number of machines and their cost make the choosing difficult for physicians who at times must make selective, godlike decisions in matters of lifesaving.

In American medicine when forces of science and activism play more significant roles than humanism, striking paradoxes occur. On one hand medical centers in the United States are the best place in the world for a human being to have a serious illness and on the other, it is difficult to obtain a physician's care or reassurance for major or minor illness in the American home.*

The activist thinking in medicine provides the best lifesaving drugs and surgical techniques but frequently, in the name of doing something, unnecessary heroic techniques are employed when patients might do better without physician intervention. In these cases there are risks of minor illness becoming overmedicated, overoperated, or overinoculated; it becomes difficult in some cases to determine whether time or intervention brought symptomatic relief. Heroic measures employed in minor illness, capable of inducing chronic anxiety and "overprotectionism" in the patients, may be justified by some practitioners on the basis: "If I do not use heroic measures someone else (meaning a more activist practitioner) will." Such attitudes within the profession imply existence of value judgments made in a cynical though realistic fashion.

age 65, who die from heart disease, would be potential candidates for cardiac replacement. (Ad Hoc Task Force Heart & Lung Inst., U.S.D.H.)

*It is generally admitted among those in government responsible for delivery of medical care to its citizens that American medicine's most flagrant and tragic failure has been in reaching the needs of the poor, especially those in minority groups, either in their homes or in clinical centers. (Statement of Dr. Roger O. Egeberg, Asst. Sec. for Health & Scientific Affairs, U. S. Dept. of H. E. W. *Med. Tribune* (Jan., 1970.)

Convincing support to these judgments is often given in the name of preventive medicine, psychology, or psychiatry. At times it is obvious that individual egotism on the part of the activist practitioner becomes the governing force in therapy. He may feel whatever he does to or for the patient becomes preferable to treatment the patient might receive down the street.

Awareness of the law enters into diagnostic and therapeutic value judgments, and errors as to seriousness of illness are within the realm of *res ipsa loquitur*.* As long as more barristers than physicians are active in structuring and administering the social order, awareness of the law in the value judgments of medicine remains potent. In a litigious society incidents, sometimes minor, which occur in the physician-patient relationship can be ruled by law as being traumatic to patients (causing grief and anguish). In these cases desire for secondary gain on the part of the patient is satisfied by monetary awards in court. Thus at times physicians, in the eyes of the law, must tread narrow paths between activistic and nonactivistic judgment both in diagnosis and treatment.

Because of modern economic and materialistic forces in society, the healing art semantically has been affected or infected by the language of economics. The severity of this infection can be judged by the inordinant amount of time, energy, and financial resources spent by organized medicine on economic issues related to delivery of medical care. To the public much of the terror of illness today refers not to illness per se but its socioeconomic implications. Economic effects of illness have been variously termed as inhumane and disastrous both financially and psychologically. Mental and physical illness has become intensified, overlaid by economic anxiety among private and charity-ward patients alike; the affluent at times become bound to the poor by economics of illness. Hospitals continue to be managed in a fashion making them the most expensive of all hotels. At times patients, especially the elderly, question the importance of their survival

---

*In recent years, there has been what organized medicine considers a crisis of "professional liability" due to the growing problem of malpractice lawsuits and rising costs of insurance to cover physicians against lawsuits.

when daily charges cause an increasing sense of financial anguish or even disaster. To date forms of "sickness insurance" (frequently misnamed "health insurance") are not totally protective or humanitarian in design, especially in light of socioeconomic complications resulting from progress and activism in American medicine.

American medicine continues (albeit with less confidence) to postulate free enterprise referable to the delivery of medical care. This in a sense denies the true nature of illness and separates it from other forms of human misery. The language of buyer and seller found in the general economic order is transposed in the healing art in its dialogue with the social order. Copostulated and transposed is the concept of choice of product on a voluntary selective basis for those who seek healing—the arms-length bargaining for value in the marketplace. Thus a concerned public has become preoccupied with health as a purchasable item.

Health is looked upon in terms of a commodity bought in the marketplace, which raises curious and paradoxical questions: How long (during the lifespan) does health and "health insurance" remain purchasable? What is the nature of the commodity being bought? Is it peace of mind, tranquility, holiness (health, whole, hale), good mastication or digestion, or reasonably regular bowel or urinary function? Should the sale of this commodity be governed by *caveat emptor* or *caveat venditor*? Does the "purchase" of health within modern context change the nature of the physician in his relationship to the patient?

Adding semantic difficulties to the discourse on health and health services are names given to insurance coverage for cost of medical care according to age and socioeconomic status of beneficiaries. Thus through fragmentation of totality the units of "omnicare" become "Medicare," "Medicaid," "Medicost," and "Medicredit."* These names represent a language of synthesis, postpone-

---

*Semantically this term is most poor and misleading. (See article "A.M.A. urges Medicredit, Voluntary Health Insurance." *Medical Tribune* (November 20, 1969.) "Medicredit" (Fulton-Broyhill bill—HR 18567) would allow tax credits for purchase of health insurance on a sliding scale with greatest relief to low income people; Federal vouchers for insurance provided for indigent; Benefit standards; peer review mechanism.

ment, and compromise in the dialogue among opposing forces of social action in American medicine.

We can see how the practice of medicine today may become a bizarre exercise in philosophy and language for the student or practitioner, no matter how dedicated. Great philosophical questions plague the practitioner seeking meanings of "purviews," "rights," and "privileges" in relationships with patients and people generally. His political beliefs may be bound to one or another opposing philosophy. To the right of his self-concept he may see himself as a conservative, without strong social commitment; to the left his alter ego makes him lean toward socialism or social action of whatever variant. As a conservative his art may become, as in the thesis of Schiller, a "mere breadearning craft." His alter ego places him in a humanitarian role, identifying him in a powerful fashion closely to all other human beings (*Agape*).

If the modern practitioner explores the true dimensions of his profession he asks, Is it an art or a science? On the basis of a personal interaction between physician and patient, can it be properly termed an art? Is personal interaction still fundamental to the physician-patient relationship in these days of great technical accomplishment in medicine?

The art of healing, based only partially on science, as yet has not become a specialized sphere of scientific knowledge. Much biomonitoring of human phenomena is done with techniques borrowed from biophysics and biochemistry. There remains a gulf separating principles in medicine and the theoretical values dealt with by those in pure basic scientific endeavors.

In diagnosis and treatment of illness medicine depends on direct adaptations of techniques used in physics or chemistry; but these cannot be applied as in physical sciences, where observations are usually complete. In medical practice practical time limits set by the need for investigation and treatment of the patient in relationship to money spent limit observation. Further, no amount of investigation or observation can reveal the clinical situation in toto; hence medical modalities are based on probabilities of a low order while those in physical and other sciences on a higher order. Experienced practitioners of the healing art know that in dealing with human beings they rely entirely on borrowed knowledge and techniques of science. Further "Basic" scientists who staff teaching hospitals know they justify their clinical presence in these institutions by only partially illuminating those dark areas of diagnosis readily accessible to ordinary clinical intuition or acumen.

The practice of medicine as an art continues to depend on the personal interaction of the physician's intuition and acumen in relation to another human being. He often must respond to cues of which he may not be fully aware. This latter quality may be termed inspiration or artful intuition.

Thus medicine borrows techniques and viewpoints of both the arts and the sciences; and as a profession its language should be consonant not with business or husbandry but with scientific and artistic dedication. This involves more than commitment to old Hippocratic principles and is guaranteed by neither law nor education. We cannot hope for a preponderence of physicians in the grand tradition of François Rabelais, priest, philosopher, and physician. We can hope for a tradition of balanced humanistic and scientific attributes in practitioners without which the profession could revert to the status of a skilled trade.

Both scientific and humanistic studies can be intellectually and spiritually satisfying to the physician.* Historically they appear to have satisfied the widely divergent intellectual tastes and creative bents of such personalities as Francis Bacon, William Harvey, August Comte, and Claude Bernard. The judicious practice of medicine would seem to require a careful blending of both studies in the education of the physician. This would give practitioners greater opportunities to communicate those ideas important to their art and to put in proper perspective techniques borrowed from biochemists and physicists. Yet graduates of medical schools today are not well grounded in the humanities. This attests to an un-

____

*Graduates in philosophy, political science, and economics are being accepted at McMaster University Medical School in Canada with only eight weeks of preparation or orientation in the language of "science." It is hoped this trial curriculum will bring to the practice of medicine versatility in background more relevant to medicine of the future. (*Medical Tribune,* April 9, 1970.)

wavering belief among educators that ultimately most future physicians will evolve as pure scientists. A whole generation of practitioners today lack communicative skills other than in diagnostic, prognostic, and therapeutic language containing biochemical overtones. Communicative skills in determining how patients feel and in obtaining the natural history of disease are becoming a lost art.

There are manifest conflicts between art and science in medicine, which create paradoxes. What is "best" scientifically to promote longevity in preterminal and terminal illness may be the worst treatment for the patient as a social being with family and community ties. The accessibility of highly scientific therapeutic modalities has proven the case for the large medical center over the home sickroom in extending lives of these patients. In medical centers terminal cases with disordered kidney function receive dialysis; those with severe anemia, blood transfusions. In cases of fungating lesions, necessary surgical debridement can be performed; those with fluid in the abdomen receive regular trocar draining.

Even with the advent of home-care units for terminal illnesses, services received by the individual at home remain inferior. While the patient at home loses in terms of longevity, the art of medicine is served in what he may gain in terms of happiness. The family may benefit in having opportunity during the pregrief periods for realistic reconciliation without much of the false hope engendered in hospital care. Visiting patients daily at some distant medical center, at times a gruesome experience, is obviated for members of the patient's family. When death does come at home, as it inevitably would in a medical center, generally the family accepts it more readily. Frequently they are better able to meet the future financially if not emotionally. Even the affluent of our society at times find the cost of institutional care in preterminal and terminal illness financially catastrophic.

The paradox described in the healing art today is a disturbing example of the gulf between benefits offered patients in a scientific sense by "noncommunity" medical centers and man's propensity toward happiness as a tribal, social, talking-to-himself,

time-binding, rational animal. Schweitzer had this in mind at La-
barann when tribal families of patients were invited to live on
hospital grounds.

Other social and economic problems have been created by
advances in surgical techniques, long before the era of organ
transplants. For some years sizable numbers of surgical and medical patients have taken residence near great medical centers to be
near unique or specialized regimens of care available in these
centers. Today those with new hearts, kidneys, lungs, eyes, ears,
and bone frequently dislocate their total life situations to receive
follow-up care. Hoped for is a future emergence of general and
specialized services available away from large clinics in smaller
communities and neighborhoods.

Heretofore bigness has been equated with excellence in the
evaluations of medical institutions. This synonymity has been true
in a scientific sense; two or three generations of practitioners have
been led away from the art in healing through awareness acquired
by early training in large medical centers. Practitioners continue
to find patients as social beings in neighborhoods unlike those with
whom they communicated in clinical clerkship, internship, and
residency training. This is understandable since human beings give
up much individuality when crossing thresholds of inpatient and
outpatient services in medical centers. This is especially true of
cases used as texts for teaching purposes.

In neighborhoods or communities patients as social beings have
expectations of medical care consonant with a status different from
that attainable in the more impersonal environment of the large
medical center. Admittedly there are perhaps insoluble or insur-
mountable obstacles to the ideal of daily compassionate, expeditious excellence in large hospitals. However in a semantic sense
it is the patient's rights and the staff's privileges that must be pre-
served. Hospital protocols should speak of patient rights and
privileges. Patients who cannot exercise their rights within the
hospital eventually may exercise them outside, politically and in
ways disturbing to the homeostasis of the profession.

Physicians may unwittingly, by language or actions, deny identity to patients as franchised citizens or social beings and forget

that patients have political or social opinions in busy clinical milieus. In hospital settings, large or small, all patients become elemosynary or "charity" cases entitled to the *caritas* and compassion of humane diagnosis and treatment procedures. Unfortunate is a language that frames at once economics, ethics, and virtue in human relationships: the words *public* and *nonpublic charge* become devoid of meaning. Nowadays most medical services within the purview of the healing art are apt, in some fashion, to be indebted to the public. Who can claim the dubious title of private patient in a hospital where the physical plant, the equipment, the trained personnel (including part of the physician's education), the research, and procedures have been paid for in whole or in part by the public?

CHAPTER I

American Medical Association News Weekly editions (1966-1969).

Billroth, T. *The Medical Sciences in the German Universities, A Study in the History of Civilization, trans.* W. H. Welch. New York: Macmillan Company, 1924.

Boehaave, Hermann. *Aphorisms Concerning the Knowledge and Cure of Disease.* (Translation from last edition printed in Latin at Leyden, 1728; with observations and explanations by A. Bettesworth and C. Hitch, London, 1735.)

Bowra, C. M. *The Greek Experience.* New York: The World Publishing Co., 1961.

Carcopino, J. *Daily Life in Ancient Rome: The People and the City at the Height of the Empire,* trans. E. O. Lorimer. New Haven: Yale University Press.

Carrington, P. *The Early Christian Church,* 2 vols. London: Cambridge University Press, 1957.

Castiglioni, A. *History of Medicine.* New York: Alfred A. Knopf, 1941.

Childe, V. Gordon. *Man Makes Himself.* New York: A Mentor Book, The New American Library, 1951-1961.

Clark, George. *Early Modern Europe.* New York: A Galaxy Book, Oxford University Press, 1960.

Cochrane, C. N. *Christianity and Classical Culture.* New York: Oxford University Press, 1952.

Davies, John Llewelyn; Vaughan, David James, trans. *The Republic of Plato.* London: MacMillan & Co. Ltd., 1943.

Dictionary of Christian Biography, W. Smith (ed.). London: J. Murray, Vol. I, p. 691, 1958.

"Dr. Alice Hamilton." *Industrial Medicine and Surgery,* 4:421, 1953. Ibid Tribute to Alice Hamilton. Amer. Journal Public Health. Feb. 1969.

Eiseley, Loren. *The Immense Journey.* New York: Random House Inc., 1962.

Garrison, F. H. *An Introduction to the History of Medicine.* Philadelphia: W. B. Saunders Co., Fourth ed., 1929.

Gondoni, G. and Longhi, R. "La Vita Dei Santi Cosmae Damiano Narrata dal Beato Angelico." *Rass. Med.,* 35:25-40 (Jan. & Feb.), 1958.

Hamilton, Edith. *The Greek Way.* New York: W. W. Norton & Co., Inc., 1942.

Hamilton, W. *History of Medicine.* London: H. Colburn and R. Bentley, 1831.

Hippocrates. "Epidemics I & II," in Hippocrates, Jones, W. H. S., Withington E. T. (Eng. translation). Vol. I London, England: W. E. Heineum, 1923, pp. 139-287.

Kelly, Howard A. *Cyclopedia of American Medical Biography*. Philadelphia: W. B. Saunders, 1912.

Keynes, G. The Oslerian Tradition. *British Medical Journal,* 2: 599, 1968.

Kitto, H. D. F. *The Greeks.* Baltimore: Penguin Books, 1961.

McCord, Gary P. *Blood Letting and Bandaging.* Arch. Environ. Health, Vol. 20, #4, April 1970.

"Medicine." One of a Series of Interviews on the American Character. Fund for the Republic, Center for the Study of Democratic Institutions, Santa Barbara, California, 1962.

Meiklejohn, A. *The Life, Work and Times of Charles Turner Thackrah* (1795-1833). Edinburgh: Livingstone, 1957.

Osler, W. *The Evolution of Modern Medicine.* New Haven: Yale University Press, 1923.

Page, Irving. Surgeons thru A Physician's Eye. *Modern Medicine,* June 30, 1969.

Paracelci (Phillipi Theophrastus Bombastus von Hohenheim). *Volume Medicinae.* Strasbourg: Briscoium, 1616.

Perrin, Noel. *Dr. Bowdler's Legacy: A History of Expurgated Books in England and America.* New York: Atheneum Press.

Ramazzini, B.; Robert Legge. *Ind. Med. and Surgery.*

Rush, Benjamin (1743?-1813) Medical Inquiries & Associations. 5 Vols. Philadelphia (1789-1798).

Russell, Bertrand. *A History of Western Philosophy.* New York: Simon and Schuster,

Sedgwick, W. T. "Foundations of Prevention." *Bull. Amer. Acad. Med.,* 11:692, 1910.

Sigerist, H. E. *On the History of Medicine.* New York: M.D. Publications, Inc., 1960.

Werner, J. *Aristotle: Fundamentals of the History of His Development,* trans. Richard Robinson. London: Oxford University Press.
(The evolution of Aristotelian scientific and philosophic doctrines, studied chronologically.)

Wilder, A. *History of Medicine,* New Sharon, Me.: New England Eclectic Publishing Co., 1901.

CHAPTER II

Semantics in the Verbal World of Health,

Disease (Cancer), and Clinical Settings

We have indicated that "health" is looked upon by many in our materialistic society as a purchasable commodity even though very few if any laymen or physicians have a true definition of the commodity. Both health and disease are relative concepts, not static entities. The relativity is one of time; i.e., phase of life of a particular human being in relation to others. Health in a positive sense has been defined as the capacity of the human organism to be *reasonably* free of undue pain, discomfort, disability, limitation of action, or social capacity. This definition is filled with value terms and semantic uncertainties. The same would be true if disease were defined in an opposite fashion. A resolution of these value terms relating to health or disease requires a unified concept of total "body" organization at all levels: biochemical, cellular, organ, interpersonal, social, and economic. This unified totality in concept of disease requires a holistic multifactor rather than a unit factor (a singular disease process) approach; it can afford both to the physician and the patient a semantically useful form of awareness in health maintenance and in the cure of disease.*

Under a unified concept of disease, pathology remains a "bad" influence to the degree it affects ability of the individual to survive threats in his internal or external environment. Lack of knowl-

---

*The author shares some of the beliefs on this subject, held by Gunnar Biorck, Serafimor Hospital, Stockholm. He believes that there are many human beings who should be encouraged to live full, productive and emotionally rich lives, regardless of potentially hazardous stressors inherent in such lives. While we are achieving marginal effects in controlling morbidity and mortality in lung, coronary, and neoplastic diseases by

edge of compensatory mechanisms in man (cellular, enzymatic, and biochemical) leads us to label all body defense mechanisms as pathological or "bad" when in truth they may be good for the individual depending upon the nature of the threat from either his internal or external environment.

An Aymara Indian living in the Andes may have a normal blood count of 8,000,000 red cells per cubic millimeter; this would be considered pathological for white men living at sea level in a temperate climate who have a "normal" red cell count of 4,500,-000 to 5,000,000. We have here an example of an adaptation of the internal environment of man in a "pathological" fashion to the external environment.

In the realm of psychiatry, patterns of behavior, anxiety states, or mania might jeopardize survival of individuals in the complexities of a large city and as such would be "bad." The same behavior patterns have different connotations in more permissive or protective environments in villages or small towns.

We must conclude that the words *norms, normal, health, disease,* and *infirmity* semantically have different meanings for different people. They define one term by opposing it to another and within different contexts of time, places, and external environmental forces at work. What we consider health is really the ability of the living organism to effect optimal adjustment to its total individual circumstances.

When medicine was emerging from much of its empiricism at the beginning of the twentieth century, its language of extramural communication had been "locked," in some respects, like that of isolated societies' speaking code understandable only to its members. Empiricism with its inherent uncertainties in ministering to the sick had fostered some obfuscation in medicine's language;*

preventive measures and regulation of health hazards, it is not always wise to interfere with special features of an individual's way of life simply to achieve longevity; especially if it causes great unhappiness and blocks fulfillment. The achievement of the goals of a "happy" life within a shorter life span (La Vida Breve), philosophically, places the whole subject of health and disease in a more balanced perspective except where "actuarial calculism" is concerned.

*Uncertainties in ministration to the sick led Voltaire in his "A Philosophical Dictionary" to characterize physicians of his day as "Men who

it also had inherited language proven utilitarian for its internal communication, and for preserving its homeostasis. A convoluted language and at times a conspiracy of silence have been used by societies of physicians* in dealing with what they considered threats from within its ranks, as in the persecution of Ignaz Semmelweis in Vienna. (See Morton Thompson, "The Cry and the Covenant," New York, Doubleday and Company, 1949.)

Words, as Freud stressed repeatedly, have impact physically and mentally on those who suffer as well as those who diagnose and treat disease. All dialogue whether it be ordinary or technical can affect the patient, the physician, and the "workings" of disease. In recent years organized medicine in the United States, through editorial educational endeavor, has developed awareness among its members relating to problems of word usage in medical technical writing. This endeavor encourages a higher standard of scientific quality and readability of material for nurses, physicians, and other interested readers. However medicine, over the years, has paid little attention to semantic reaction hazards (of health) to patients or the public generally when members of the profession employ ordinary, quasi-technical, and technical language in either the written or spoken word.

Most professions and trades have "private" technical languages, often intelligible only to initiates. The shorthand communication of hospital or clinic milieus, a far cry from the language of Hippocrates, has become a modern necessity in exchange of medical information among nurses, physicians; also for those responsible for pious accountancy of clinical procedure.

Though utilitarian, terms such as *B.U.N.* (descriptive of patients' blood urea nitrogen content) can in the patient's mind demean the dignity of his bodily function. While fully significant to the clinician, such descriptive brevity may impart to the patient a feeling that his "life's blood" and for that matter his blood-forming organs are being regarded too casually. As a noninitiate

prescribe medicines of which they know little, to cure diseases of which they know less, in human beings of whom they know nothing." Earlier this viewpoint was sarcastically portrayed by Molière in the play "Le Médecin Malgré Lui" and in "Le Malade Imaginaire."

*Gesellschaft der Aerzte Vienna (Society of Physicians).

he to a degree can become alienated or feel left out when descriptive brevity is spoken in his presence. Often, what the profession considers acceptable language on the ward is based on the assumption that only initiates hear or understand it. Restriction of audience today is difficult; and modern patients are "health educated" and knowledgeable more so than at any time in the history of medicine. Some patients are able, during long periods of hospitalization, to commit to memory B.U.N.'s, the R.B.C.-W.B.C. Shilling Index, and a variety of often repeated clinical laboratory determinations. He may learn to recite his life history verbatim as detailed on clinical charts. Hospital staffs on specialty rounds gather about these "learned" patients, absorbed in technical shorthand, at times ignore questions such as "Doctor, why do I still hurt here?" or, "Do I have to have another 'procedure'?" In this manner the patient's feeling of alienation increases and an already damaged ego becomes further traumatized.*

The profession also has invented shorthand combinations of words, often jargon, which impart false meaning. Words like "cardiac diet" refer not to the heart but to persons who have heart disease and to physiological complications of that disease. Brevity produces no meaning in the words "obesity pill" since the term is nondescriptive of either a curative, anticipatory, or preventive modality. False awareness created by such expressions is not merely grammatical but one of false knowledge.

In considering the impact of language pertaining to health, we must realize that while there are many lay persons with superior knowledge and analytical abilities, most cannot evaluate evidence given by medical authors writing in a popular style on health subjects ranging from rheumatism to hypokinetic disease. Often, as a result of purposeful constriction in scope of subject and lack of critical insight on the part of the reader, these writings impart a

*It is a credit to the sensitivity of those hospital administrators in more "charitable" teaching institutions that patients are spared this traumatic experience by requiring that pertinent clinical data not be discussed in the patient's presence. Ego-smashing mass onslaughts of palpating and auscultating by grimacing physicians and students are avoided. Language of reinforcement and reassurance is routine no matter how grave the state of illness, and science is not advanced at the expense of humane conduct.

false sense of medical acumen in the reader; further, they may induce *hypochondriasis* and *iatrogenesis* (fear of disease and physician-induced disease).

Perhaps there is no greater pestilence than the excessive spread of information and misinformation on health subjects, much of which is widely distributed in a free press long before it can be critically and fully evaluated; its language is seductive and panaceic. Those buying or reading such material do so to "learn," not to evaluate. Misrepresentations in labeling or advertising of medications are quickly cured by government regulation. However at times miasmic volatilization of baseless statements on health go unchallenged and are accepted as revelation simply because they appear in a printed document. Neighborhood consultation groups, using these materials as bibles, advise each other *ex cathedra* on problems ranging from sexual intercourse in marriage to the relationships of catecholamines in exercise tolerance. With each succeeding perversive—and successful—edition, more and more persons are drawn into varied forms of health cultisms. Medical misinformation is not easily curtailed; freedom of the press guarantees the right of the public to analyze and judge the value of any printed product. While sources of health misinformation are by no means limited to physician authors, we must suspect that they arose in a vacuum of information partially due to the impersonal mode of modern medical practice.

Published true information on health also has been shown to produce hypochondriasis and to be potentially iatrogenic. We must add that the manner in which physicians label ailments of patients, physical and mental, can in a semantic sense also be iatrogenic. Patients usually have no knowledge of disease entities in a formal sense prior to the experience of diagnosis or treatment. They are aware first of disease in an informal sense by not feeling well or knowing that "things" are not "working" properly, but without knowledge of import of symptoms. Thus they speak first a language of symptomatology to which the ego becomes attuned; then when "labeled" with a specific illness, patients speak a different language and develop different self-concepts. How symptomatology is translated by the physician into descriptive pathology or in some other way more consonant with disordered function, determines important semantic reactions in the patient. Descriptive classification of pathology and disease identification certainly are necessary to the physician. However in physical illness, and much more so in mental illness, the descriptive abnormal physiology of disease (disordered function) is more consonant with what the patient already has experienced and frequently it is less traumatic; at times more beneficial to him. Patients frequently understand and adjust better to being told why and how "things" are not "working" than being told they have *thrombocytopenic purpura* or *Hyperosmolarity.* This concept is not new to those in psychiatry who frequently must bring to patients an understanding of why they act in a certain manner within aspects of their total life situations; this is fundamental to rehabilitative efforts in mental illness. A great deal of the efficacy in healing by Christian Science methods is based on this important concept.

No discussion of the verbal world of disease would be complete without consideration of semantic reactions, attitudes, and behavior of human beings brought face to face with the most unfortunate word in the medical lexicon, "cancer." There are other diseases which, at times, are fatal or hopeless (forms of coronary disease, advanced pulmonary tuberculosis, disseminated lupus erythematosis); the semantic reactions induced by these diseases usually do not produce the enormous difficulties in the world of words, attitudes, behavior as those produced by the diagnosis of cancer.

To analyze semantic reactions we must first look to the cultural folklore or mythological matrix in which the word "cancer" became imbedded. This matrix lay in the hidden "Permian" foundation of language mentioned earlier in the book, where the fossilization or embalmment of meaning and concepts occur during human history. In this fashion cancer—crab of the zodiac of ancient astrologers and astronomers—forms the "bedrock" of a mysterious world of events.* On this bedrock structure is superimposed the world of the oncologists (pathologists) and their

*In the hidden world of propositions and doctrines it is of interest semantically to speculate the impact of Boerhaave's *Aphorisms,* had he emphasized the likeness of the "schirrus" to asparagus or seaweed.

doctrinal theories, propositions, macroscopic and microscopic observations, and tabulations of data. Another level of events or happenings occurs at even higher strata in this language structure; these are what we will call specialist views of the cancer world: the urologist who sees cancer of the prostate; the surgeons who see cancer of the breast, lung, uterus, or colon; and the dermatologist who sees cancer of the skin—even the psychiatrist who sees in the patient the threat of progressive destruction of body ego.

The bias of specialized views emerges with its own language; and with or without the general practitioner, acting as intermediate or the patient's advocate, the word cancer is introduced into the logical everyday world of events of the patient, his family, and his friends. Regardless of the location and nature of the diagnosed tumor, cancer is cancer to most patients and their intimates. This is true regardless of proven success in treatment and outlook for patients with a particular type of tumor; in the word world, cancer is cancer; i.e., an eating away of flesh, and there is a feeling of hopelessness for the patient (many times by the physician) and his intimates. In continuing the unqualified use of the word cancer (for a variety of organs affected) in the disease world, Uncle George's cancer of the prostate, with its one well-circumscribed or walled-off nodule, produces the same semantic reaction as the late Aunt Martha's cancer of the breast, which "spread and spread." When the specialist or general practitioner expresses optimism in the case of Charlie's skin cancer which was removed, Charlie's family or friends may still think of the optimism voiced by the physician of Alberta, the green grocer's wife, now long gone from this world; she had a cancer "somewhere" in her uterus. Thus through too common usage, the word cancer equates and projects much which is "bad" in tumor pathology, regardless of nature and extent of organ involvement. Its use by the most conscientious public and private agencies, in their health education media, though noble and well-intentioned, seeks purposely through alarmist methods to detect early or cure or prevent the disease. The verbal world of these agencies, which may intrude in the midst of the playing of a Brahms symphony over the radio, is a constant reminder to the author, for one, that a semantic refurbishment is required in the "world" of neoplastic diseases; this applies mainly to those strata of its events and happenings that semantically affect the constricted awareness of the ordinary, untutored, uninitiated man on the street.

In looking at possible solutions to language and concomitant attitude and behavior problems related to the broad usage of the word cancer, it will facilitate matters first to diagram what we have already considered on this subject. Diagram analogy, employing strata, must be looked upon in the same light as geologic formations of the earth, where various layers remain hidden except when fractured convolutions in the earth's crust cause what geologists term a "show," which presents to the viewer the cross-sectional (usually partial) anatomy of the earth's surface.

Logic "dictates" that we begin at the bottom of the figure we construct and build upward to that word world which we will name "the happy hills of home," with rolling green terrain undisturbed except by the rumination of farmers and lowing cattle. We are not however concerned here with the precise logic of seismology, mathematics, or physics; we are merely borrowing a structural map from geology to explore a problem in awareness and general semantics. So we shall begin at the top, where the word cancer, like an unheralded new volcano, has erupted on a peaceful and happy landscape of human events.

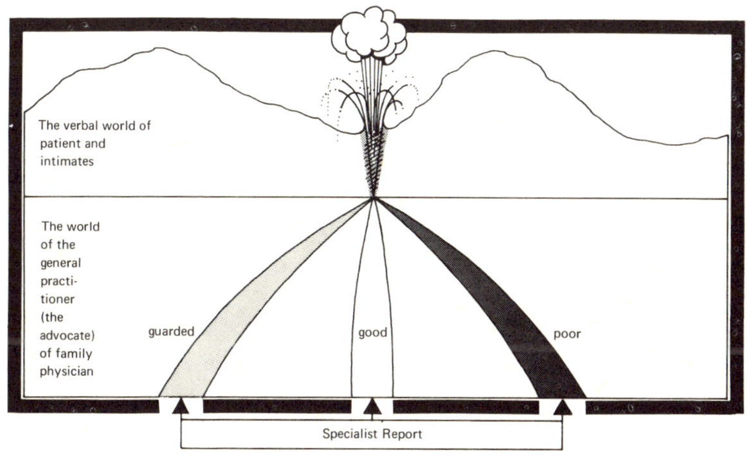

We note in this stage of the diagram that what appeared on the peaceful surface in the lives of the patient and his intimates was being fed by a triumverate of possibilities in outlook (prognosis), where meaning of specialist reports was transmitted to the patient or his family. In this transmission by the patient's advocate, or family physician, the physician, depending upon his reaction to the disease entity, may or may not have, through either symbolic or verbal language, colored (through his own darker or lighter awareness) the specialist report on talking to the patient or the family.

So far we have charted strata of words, events, and happenings where meaning and semantic impact of the word cancer has remained somewhat uniform and close to the surface of the world of health education, the news media, the everyday world of

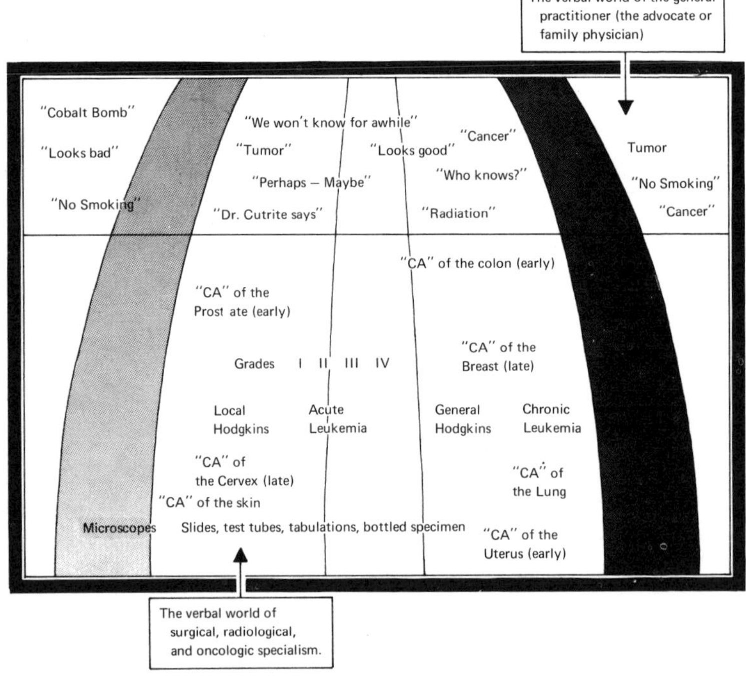

people who have known other people with the disease. Though this area of reaction is close to the surface, it is no less black or isolating for the person who bears the name "cancer patient."

Since it was "that specialist's report" that made the cancer patient, in a sense, a marginal human being, we must somehow explore the deeper strata of events—a more hidden and more mysterious doctrinal and propositional world of specialized techniques and observations. It was from this specialized awareness that the report of outlook or prognosis for the patient emanated.

We find in this diagram all the uncertainties, complexities of diagnosis, prognosis, and treatment in cancer pathology, which is mainly a verbal world relatively unintelligible to the untutored and uninitiated. As mentioned, however, it is from this stratum that cancer, regardless of what stage in development and in what organ, that the impact or semantic reaction at the top of the diagram (the verbal world of patients and intimates) is mainly fed. Thus the word cancer applied at this level semantically tends to equate all tumor pathology, regardless of whether the prognosis is good, poor, or guarded. Thus an early well-circumscribed non-etastatic cancer of the prostate, or an extirpated suspicious polyp of the colon (both with good prognoses) semantically become

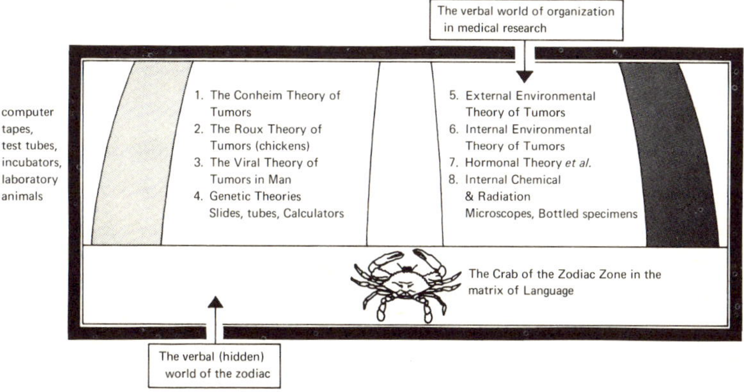

verbally equated, through the use of the word cancer, with metastatic breast or other highly malignant tumors.

We have two more strata in our geological diagram to consider. These are close to bedrock and pertain to extremes; i.e., man the discoverer, inventor, and scientific investigator and man who has remained during a conspectus of millions of years in his history influenced by signs, symbols, Totemism, and mythology.

These structures were superimposed to emphasize the indomnitable spirit of mankind, which refuses to submit to fears of the unknown. It is from these structures that hope and progress in conquest of malignancies have evolved, though they remain yet in the Permian formation of the hidden world of cancer. There is hope that even before the crab of the zodiac is removed as a threat to the body ego of men that its name, Cancer, will disappear from the language of pathology—not all tumors regardless of degree and extent of malignancy need be termed cancer. When this refurbishment in language occurs, perhaps there will be less anguish in those "happy hills of home" for those with tumor pathology with excellent prognoses who now suffer the leprosy of diagnosis. In our society a tremendous amount of talent or competence is being spent on "language" and "intuitive" processes of machines in computer technology. Surely there are those in this talented group, with skill in linguistics or philology, capable of solving some of the problems in the verbal world of human beings. Perhaps when these talents are put to use by the healing art, we can eliminate from its lexicon words such as *cancer, malignancy,* and unfortunate language such as *heart attacks* (who is the attacker?) and *homes for incurables.*

To examine further verbal, nonverbal, and symbolic dialogue between modern patients and physicians we must look carefully at those elements in the relationship, both conscious and unconscious, which each *brings* to the scene of the clinical examination setting. Much that is brought to the clinical scene by both physician and patient is not pure expression of free will but mixture or fusion of ambivalent ideas and expectations.

The physician brings *what* he is in terms of symbolic authoritarianism along with those conscious and unconscious uncertainties based on his memories of past ministrations. The physician also brings a listening process whereby he understands and evaluates words and symptoms of the patient in terms of his own awareness and even his own problems and perhaps those of his loved ones.

Practitioners of the healing art, whether they be physicians or dentists, particularly the most dedicated and conscientious, subject themselves sooner or later in life to a continuing process of self-analysis. This process is related to their professional life spectrum with its successes and failures. The physicians who have seen the same group of patients for a long period of time may suffer from *scrupulosity* (sometimes a feeling of hopelessness) and wonder if the medical results, seen later in the lives of their patients, could have been better had different decisions been made earlier. These feelings or attitudes of doubt unfortunately appear strongest among physicians approaching the winter of professional life. These feelings are affected as much by the physician's age as that of his patients. Their counterparts in the dental profession may become even more discouraged since these prime healers must view directly in the mouths of their older and devoted patients the results hearkening back to days when old deficiencies in dental technology defeated judgments and efforts of the best and most dedicated dental practitioners.

All these events and happenings occurring in the personal world of the practitioner, medical or dental, usually remain hidden to the patient. Nonetheless they play important roles in patient relationships in clinical settings.

The patient brings to the examination setting not only his physical symptoms but a striving for emotional safety by maintaining some semblance of balance or fusion between those forces of love and aggression within him. He has expectations (aside from medical technical competence) concerning the physician's availability, unhurried attention, and compassion. Barriers of time and an unrelaxed physician office routine can become symbolic semantic obstructions to these expectations.

How the patient responds to the language of the physician may, to a significant degree, be determined by what prior experience he may have had with authority figures: a father or a boss who was too strict a disciplinarian, a minister who frowned on him, a policeman who was rude; or he may have been treated with lack of compassion by a physician in military service. The physician as an authority figure accentuates this role by asking the patient intimate questions, telling him to undress, and by thumping, pounding, and probing during the medical examination. Overlying verbal and symbolic dialogue in the clinical setting is the modern cultural pattern of relationships between physician and patients. Physicians routinely ask questions and instruct the patients to undress. Further, in our culture physicians examine patients completely, a procedure most persons will never allow anyone else to perform. So what is routine and standard procedure for male and female patients goes unquestioned. Forgotten, but of semantic import, is the fact that in many clinical confrontations *a* particular patient may never have been examined by *a* particular physician, and the experience for both is unique.

Patients speak a body language influenced by the degree to which they experience infantilization or regression in the clinical setting. Also, those who clutch the table or their garments speak a language to the physician, telling him their fears of either the examination or exposure of self-concept as a miserable physical specimen. The body speaks with a muscle rigidity, a dry mouth, moist palms, as expression of anxiety. During anxiety patients verbalize ideas appropriate or inappropriate to the clinical setting. In this random language patients seek reassurance either by word or in the mood and manner of the physician.

Demands upon physicians in conducting a dialogue of compassion, support, or reassurance are in proportion to degree of patient sensitization to clinical examination procedures and to the particular kinds of abnormalities disclosed by the examination. When a physician emphasizes the finding of a good strong heartbeat to a patient, he may overcome some of the patient's infantalized feelings and some of the emotional trauma connected with defect discovery. At the conclusion of clinical evaluations the physician's language can further infantalize the patient or induce undue anxiety in him, depending on the patient's life situation, age, occupation, and already existing fears and phobias. Here, the friendly image of the physician may prove to be useful in patient reassurance especially if he stresses in a sincere and complimentary manner normal examination findings in relationship to abnormalities detected. If he lacks a friendly father image, he may by his mood and manner aggravate further the patient's life situation over and above his concern for his physical defect or illness. In such unfortunate instances of clinical confrontations the meeting between patient and healer can be both a scientific success and a miserable failure in the exercise of artful intuition in healing.

CHAPTER II

Boehaave, Hermann. Aphorisms on the Knowledge and Cure of Disease. Translation from last edition printed in Latin at Wexdon, 1728 (Osby Bettesworth & Hibbs, London, 1735).

Bois, J. Samuel. *Communications and Creative Experience,* Viewpoints Inst. Inc., Los Angeles, California, 1965.

Bois, J. Samuel. *Exploration in Awareness.* New York: Harper & Row, 1957.

Ibid. *The Art of Awareness.* Dubuque, Iowa: W. C. Brown Co., 1966.

Current Concepts in Management of Cancer. Bulletin, Southern Medical Assoc. Vol. 57, No. 1, March 1969.

Engle, George L. *A Unified Concept of Health and Disease In Life and Disease,* Dwight J. Ingle (ed.). New York: Basic Books, 1963.

Levin, Lowell S. *Building Toward the Future—Implications for Health Education.* Anresbur. Public Health Vol. 519., No. 11, November 1969.

May, Jacques M. *The Ecology of Human Disease.* New York: M.D. Publications, 1958.

Menninger Clinic Seminars. Menninger Clinic, Topeka, Kansas (1962).

Root, Maurice T. *The Aging M.D. and His Practice.* Medical Opinion Review, Vol. 5, No. 11, November 1969.

CHAPTER III

The Education and Self-Concept of the Physician

Within a New Philosophy of Medicine

We see the present state of the healing art leaning heavily, for a theoretical basis and language, on physics, chemistry, biology. While physicians of other centuries made humanities and philosophy part of wisdom, there seems to have been insufficient time for modern medicine to develop a firm interest in either because of its dynamic technical achievement. New theories and techniques borrowed daily from chemistry, physics, genetics, and other biological sciences add large increments of knowledge and modalities. There has been little time for exploring general philosophic implications of these modalities or the economics of delivering new services to human beings.

The art of healing requires a philosophical basis to begin with; it has within itself historically proven possibilities in contributing to the general body of knowledge in philosophy (metaphysics, ontology, and cosmology). In this it has failed because of constrictions placed on the art by latter-day medical educators and passed onto modern generations of physicians. Medical educators who explore confusion surrounding the purpose of medical schools face conflicting interests in their own ranks; there are inherent academic prejudices or priorities toward one form or another specialism (in basic science and clinical subjects). Added to the confusion are stentorian voices of researchists who control funded research. Researchists are the power and the glory of medical training institutions. Pride of authorship, not patients or teaching ability, is basic to the ego of these scientists; they have been able to inspire multitudes of young people who come into their sphere of awareness or influence. This is attested to by larger numbers of students who have chosen doctoral studies in biological physical sciences and smaller numbers who apply to medical schools.

Few modern medical educators show courage in conviction that the primary function of medical schools is to train physicians not scientists; professional humanitarians not technicians. Most, paradoxically, espouse holistic concepts of man and his psychosocial complexities but devote increasing amounts of curricular time to the purely technical and scientific aspects of medical education. Confluence of reason in medical education does not occur readily for lack of a general philosophy in the healing art, applicable or committed to a multitude of social and cultural problems existing in the world today.

A philosophy suitable for meeting the needs of various existing social and cultural problems requires that professional associations or societies of physicians possess a true modern awareness of these problems and their own self-concepts as healers, as they deal with economic and other aspects of their contractural relationships with society. A segment of leadership in medicine persists in beliefs, which in the public mind present an image or concept of omnipotence and "selfness"; this is detrimental to a reputation of practitioners for capability and sensitivity in matters of social commitment or action.

The physician's professional self-concept has been hampered in development particularly during the last fifty years for lack of basic philosophy in the teaching of medicine. In a vacuum often bereft of philosophical guidance from teachers, students of medicine recently have assumed leadership in pointing ways along paths of knowledge they feel important in curricular training. They attempt to regulate input by advising the faculty what they wish and do not wish to hear. Many students have limited interests and, as would be expected in the untrained, a constricted awareness of the healing art. At times students with limited interests and awareness have become vociferous and compelling influences in design of curricula. Faculty output narrowed to the particular interests of a given class of students can prove insufficient in scope for the training of physicians either as humanitarians or scientists.

Self-determination of curriculum by students,* though a remarkable phenomenon in the evolution of the healing art, has implications that could be productive of either fortunate or unfortunate end results. True, philosophical default in leadership by organized medicine and medical educators was brought to light by those creative minorities (the students), but techniques they propose are still unproven as successful responses in maintaining the integrity of medical practice both as an art and a science. Success or failure of these techniques or responses depends on preconceived philosophies, awarenesses, and most important, motivations students bring to a school of medicine from prior life experiences and schooling. What the student brings with him from his life prior to entering medical school is important to his hopes, aspirations, or goals and to his outlook on the educative process generally.

The desire of young men to study medicine is difficult to analyze since it may be based on both conscious and unconscious motivation. Some have in mind untimely deaths among family, friends, or relatives and may unconsciously seek a forestalling of their own untimely death. Or at the conscious level they wish powers to save the human race from what young men especially consider the "tragedy" of illness, disability, and death (love of mastery). Heroic stances of this sort frequently are converted into interest in research but more frequently into surgical specialization. Fewer physicians (unless they be physicians' daughters or sons) today are motivated to study medicine by the example of a kindly authoritarian figure of a family physician they knew in childhood and youth. Many young men hope for better future social and economic placement within society through the study of medicine and bring with them attitudes closely linked with their personal situations when they enter the study of medicine. Regardless of where the emphasis may lie, most students have important though varying degrees of altruism in motivation and

---

*New curricula in a few medical schools provide various levels of special and elective studies; students may select a variety of educational experiences.

look upon the study of medicine as a mission or calling in life. They may see little of these values to remind them of their mission on entrance to a modern medical school; neophyte students can become emotionally traumatized or disillusioned early by Academia's symbolic language of arrangement. On those early days, which should be given over to contemplation of vocation, students deal with an inordinate amount of communications surrounding costs and object orientation spoken by the establishment.

At first, cost consciousness of living expenses, books, laboratory and cadaver fees become overwhelming preoccupations and in some, productive of rut behavior. Later, obstacles to academic goals appear on the horizon in the form of basic-science hurdles. Students must learn early to plan with acumen and a great deal of pragmatism if they wish to surmount language and curricular barriers, which may block progress toward goals. When gifted with sensitivity for things as they are rather than the way they appear, neophytes learn early the prevailing supersedence of the mechanics of the educational system over its real purpose. Values in medical education become obscure even in the minds of those educators who pronounce them, daily and publicly.

Modern deans and medical educators are well versed in language of budgets, bookkeeping, and financial controls.* They, like other administrators in human society, can become too self-protective; some give inordinate attention to monitoring administrative detail, at times to the detriment of the welfare of those administered. Affairs related to the physical plant of a medical teaching institution may supersede interest in human resources. In this milieu the word "class" is emptied of meaning in the sense of its individual constituency. Students without sufficient philosophical resources, training, or guidance become strangely orientated: books assume importance beyond actual content; examinations are paramount to knowledge. Later, in clinical "clerkships," attention given clinical charts, whatever their worth, may exceed

*Medical deanships are beginning to lose their attraction for highly dedicated physicians and educators caught up in what they consider "big business," particularly those experiencing an erosion of authority due to imbalances of power resulting from structures created within medical schools and centers by federal research financing.

or supersede attention given human beings whose names appear on the chart.

In protest against some of the impersonal relationships established by the faculties and their lack of successful responses to new challenges in medical education, a determined, restless, creative minority of medical students has risen.* These are bent upon creating a modern medical philosophy, changing institutions and their rules long considered inviolate. Like younger counterparts in undergraduate education, modern medical students reject much of the political and economic status quo. Some have been alienated from western cultural values and ethical systems. Many have had no favorable authoritarian example or image of the kindly old-fashioned physician who cares *(caritas)*. They find lacking a symbolism of arrangement in the medical school conducive to the engrafting of the *caritas* concept in medical training. This refers not only to curricular matters, but to personal relationships with faculty members.

Where communication blocks with faculty occur latent feelings of alienation and anonymity are reinforced among students; these may be akin to childhood experiences. Modern faculties often have their greatest shortcomings in communicating values or philosophies, which sensitive serious-minded students feel important. A gap in interest is thus created: creative minorities among students attempt to fill the void with techniques and responses of their own; through organization they become dominant in the affairs of medical education. When their techniques prove success-

---

*Medical school administrators are now fully aware of student criticism of curricula and examinations and faculty relationships. There has been reluctance to abandon, wholesale, the old for the new. It is the administrators not the students who are held responsible for end results of radical curricula changes, as reflected in state licensing examinations and other criteria measuring quality of medical education. This responsibility could become especially onerous if succeeding graduating classes of particular medical schools had high percentages of failures in licensing examinations. So, though there may be trumpeting of change, as Dean Rogers of Johns Hopkins once expressed, "medical schools have twisted knobs a bit in altering curricula," but there has been no dramatic revision of medical education such as that which followed the Flexuer Report. See Rogers, David E. "A Dean's List of Proposals." *Medical Opinion and Review,* (October), 1969.

ful, these are passed on (mimeses) to educators. Student organizations, representing creative minorities, through the process of mimesis, already have stimulated evolution of new techniques and responses, which show promise in narrowing social distances among them; the faculty; and with those human beings who become case studies in medical teaching institutions.

In the evolutionary process taking place in medical education, significant blows have been dealt to didactic systems of lectures, held inviolate in medical education since the Middle Ages. Under didactic systems, output of faculty lecturers over the years far exceeded intake, resulting in conditions unfavorable to active intellectual growth of students. They became passive participants in the learning process. Many students still find the most they can salvage from didactic systems are bits of knowledge that each student may consider his own "hundred pearls of wisdom." These he may list in a small black notebook, one for each course of study, carefully indexed for ready reference in preparation for examinations. While he may have gained little from lectures in general understanding of magnesium metabolism, he may know the twentieth most important cause of magnesium deficiency in the human body.

Overly didactic systems of medical teaching have proven futile attempts in creating passive learning processes. Under these systems medical students in the United States can recite by rote all the mechanics, signs, and symptoms of various obstetrical presentations and yet know nothing of the social or community aspects of pregnancy among unwed mothers.* Creative minorities of students are keenly sensitive to the deficiencies and social distances involved in didactic systems; they wish changes made both in teaching techniques and curricula. Multiple tracks or pathways have been proposed to allow differentiation of interests and active pursuit of particular interests among groups of students. There is insistence among students in bringing greater family or community awareness into the curricula early in medical learning. More

*The author has found among medical students and physicians in Ireland, Scotland, and England greater awareness of various cultural milieus and social agencies; this is attributed not to medical education but to "upbringing."

confrontation with living human beings is desired* in preference to what students consider inordinate amounts of time spent in basic sciences, especially that devoted to cadaver dissection in anatomical studies.

Medical education historically has emphasized (in a chronological sense) the wrong end of life's spectrum in early medical education. The Vesalian system of anatomical study, borrowing from Aristotelian logic, proposes that the dead were once living *ergo* study of the dead will lead to knowledge of the living. In a logical, structural, or anatomical sense the proposal certainly has validity but in semantic context it is questionable. Cadavers** speak symbolic language of death to young students before learning "anatomy" of the living or much of life in an existential sense except through book learning. The language, traumatic to more sensitive individuals, speaks of medieval lore steeped in grave robbing and body snatching;*** to some students payment of cadaver fees becomes even more traumatic. To place *De Fabricus Anatomicus Humanis* in the early medical curriculum, therefore, may be logical but not always in the best interests of the students' semantic awareness.

Semantically some benefit would be derived at first from anatomical studies of the living or perhaps making these studies part of anthropology (cultural and physical) so as to foster early

*Opposed to this desire is the development of computer "patients," where computers are programmed to represent real patients with specific diseases, medical histories, and clues to their "personalities." This system propounds active participation by students in later confronting real patient problems, allowing them to diagnose and treat ailments and to learn of their mistakes. The student would continue to deal with problems as programmed, on a trial and error basis, until he satisfies the computer as to the accuracy of his diagnosis and treatment. (*Internal Medicine News,* December 1969).

**Of semantic interest is a recent proposal that the word "cadaver" be discarded in the interest of promoting favorable publicity among the public in a drive to solve donation shortages of *human dead* for use as teaching material in anatomical studies. Hoped for, through public relations techniques, is a conversion of shortage into adequacy or even a surplus under what would be termed an "anatomical gift program."

***William Burke and William Hare in Edinburgh, Scotland (1792-1829) smothered victims in order to sell human bodies for dissection, hence the word "burke"; i.e. to smother or suffocate (to murder by).

among students a holistic and historical awareness of human beings. Students then would be prone to relate early in medical learning to the whole conspectus of mankind socially, culturally, and historically. This awareness later could be productive of a more useful clinical language in settings where social distances become narrowed. Both language and self-concept of the student would benefit; his mood and manner would be less apt to impress patients as being cynical or even ghoulish. Chronic cases who visit outpatient clinics would be less apt to be termed "crocks," or those on back wards "those poor bastards on Ward A."

Relatively few licensed physicians learn as students that communications with patients often are beyond the scope of grammar or logic, sometimes beyond verbal expression. In a semantic sense, the physician's language *acting upon himself* must confront patients or other human beings whose own (as well as the physician's) language *acts upon them*. Often this complexity in communication is basis for the great number of patients who fail to comply with instructions in both the symbolic and nonsymbolic language of clinical confrontation. This is especially true when clinical language, though logical, is too formal or rejecting, too uncooperative, too authoritative, too permissive, too nonfeeling, too informative; when communications lack feedback from patient to physician.

Related to the complexities of clinical communications is the symbolic language of position or arrangement; i.e., where physicians sit or stand in relation to the patient. Even arrangement of furniture (acrossness versus alongsideness) may affect communications. Also short or long white clinical coats, while cloaking self-concepts of students, physicians, or teachers, at times can act symbolically as barriers of arrangement in communication. White uniforms play increasingly obstructive roles in communication in the healing art in proportion to increasing numbers of professionals other than physicians who wear them (barbers, cosmeticians*). Higher priorities given to basic scientific studies both at undergraduate and graduate levels of medical educa-

*A host of others: traffic wardens, cricket referees, and bakery deliverymen.

tion heretofore precluded necessary training in sensitivity and the communicative skills mentioned as part of either premedical or medical curricula. As a result of this humanistic deficit in medical education, "para-medical"* (nurses *et al.*) and other disciplines have filled these hiatuses or vacuums by practicing these skills.

Organized groups of students in some medical schools have influenced faculties to recognize the humanistic deficit in medical education. Thus some students follow the Ramazzini-Virchow precept of making humanistic or social awareness equal in importance to physiologic or pathologic awareness in their training. What students may lose in reduced study of anatomy, histology, pathology, biochemistry, and physiology may be mainly the tremendous trivia of these sciences,** soon erased after schooling from the student's armamentarium of knowledge. Some which is retained may prove ignorance as new theories evolve daily; new theories are not always extensions of older knowledge but likely to be in conflict with past knowledge.

Semantic impact of professorial titles*** among medical studies also requires consideration in relation to the student's learning process. Professorial titles tend to fragment totality and cause separatism in awareness of the healing art. Students unable to delineate boundaries of usefulness among theories and data in the basic sciences and clinical studies often become preoccupied with a quantitative input. Input may vastly exceed ability to correlate interlocking curricula data; extreme preoccupation with

---

*This term now encompasses medical "advocates," "ombudsmen," medical assistants, aides, and technicians in medical and social sciences.

**Various suggestions have been made to reform teaching the basic sciences. Some educators recognize that there are college students who enter medical school well prepared in these sciences and need little further study at graduate level. This would appear to make a strong case for study of basic sciences at college level. The use of multitrack systems (giving more basic science to some) mentioned elsewhere in this text has proven cumbersome and expensive.

***Freud, for one, opposed the "Hierarchy of Titles" prevalent in the faculty of the University of Vienna as a political and nefarious influence on medical education in that city. See Ernest Jones, *Life and Work of Sigmund Freud,* New York: Basic Books, Inc., Vol. I. 1953.

one subject may obscure its connections with interlocking theories and axioms of subjects. In this regard, arrangement of professorial titles, making all teachers in medical schools professors of the healing art, may be useful, semantically, in medical education. Teachers of anatomy and biochemistry would become healing art professors; i.e., body structure and body chemistry respectively.

Freed from imprisonment of narrow labels in specialized fields, faculty members would present greater clinical interface and could more easily identify with a totality in concept of the healing art. This could stimulate change in self-images and language more in conformity with the total learning process of students. Affected semantically too would be highly departmentalized faculty systems of teaching. Perhaps the largest and most forceful symbolic barriers of arrangement in medical education are found in these systems. Communication deadlocks can occur between departments of the faculty.

Desire for homeostasis in departments of the faculty often converts pleas for interdepartmental cooperation into threats affecting security of departments involved. Under rigid departmentalized arrangements, deans and faculty committees may argue and weigh relative values of curricular time in terms of geriatrics versus pediatrics, cardiology versus immunology, biochemistry versus anatomy. A totality in concept of the healing art becomes fragmented and lost for lack of a governing philosophy in teaching and because of vested interests of faculty departments. From this divisiveness, overriding partisan decisions are made in curricular matters favoring more influential departments over the less influential. Decisions handed down "from above" to the students heretofore made for little student participation in decision making in curricular affairs.

Of late faculty members have been interested in the voice of the student although unfortunately at times with hope of guiding students along paths of thinking favorable to one or the other department. The attitude of medical educators toward student organizations generally has, in the past, been one of tolerance. However student committees in medical schools are effecting a mimesis among educators, conducive to the attainment of larger, more valuable goals in medical education. These larger goals (sociological) have philosophical implications in the training of physicians since they contain partial solutions to existing major semantic blocks between physicians and the social order.

The language and ethical focus of the physician has been, since Hippocrates, mainly that of concern for what is good for the individual patient and the alleviation of his suffering. This is in contrast to language and ethical focus of the social order, which in its evolution is one of concern for the good of every individual collectively in society (summum bonum). The physician is conditioned by present training to observe human living matter operating within individuals biologically as opposed to those factors in human beings that operate at a social level. Because of individual patient one-to-one orientation in training, students or physicians frequently are able to relate their efforts more easily to individual good than to social good.

Larger and more valuable goals in medicine require a philosophy with more dynamic ethical focus to effect a balance between the physician's concern for individuals as biologically organized entities and concern for their equally important identities as part of an evolving social order. This implies need for changes in the kinds of physicians trained in medical schools. They may emerge in the future less trained in mechanisms of human biological organization but more broadly educated in awareness of human needs in the realm of the social order where medical services are delivered.

In examining further the profession's preparation in education for greater works, we find semantic problems in full utilization of human resources in medical education. Involved are organized self-concepts of full-time educators contrasted to part-time teachers, who volunteer valuable time from active practices to teach.

Often, a full-time educator's ideas about himself and his abilities as a teacher or administrator do not agree with disorganized images of him in the minds of students or fellow faculty members. While the full-time educator may be designated as "head" of his department, he may have few if any true disciples; though he considers himself an authority on macromolecules he may lack this recognition among colleagues. Thus organized self-concepts of full-time educators, like anyone else, may be at odds with what other individuals think of them. This is true for part-time educators as well; they may have self ideas of bravery (I compete with colleagues in private practice), patient endearment, humanitarianism, excellent professional and personal accomplishment; these self ideas may be at odds with what full-time educators, students, and colleagues generally may think of him. What he sees clearly in himself as bravery, humanitarianism, and excellence in professional or personal accomplishment may be viewed not as bravery or humanitarianism but economic endeavor; not endearment but toleration; and similar distortions.

Communicative deadlocks occur when self-concepts come under attack; these deadlocks are disruptive at a time when medical education requires full utilization of all its human resources in teaching. These disruptions occur in a few medical schools to an extent that at times jeopardizes effective teaching programs and their acceptance by students. It becomes potentially a problem in varying degrees in most if not all medical schools.

Students aware of larger, more valuable goals for medical education become cynical in attempts to understand some of the relationships of faculty members to each other. They find it difficult to rationalize conflicts among these groups of adults, men and women, selected because of common interests to be brought through similar educational experiences. Students see these same grown-up professional men and women, who after nine years of companionship in the learning process seek different, special, narrow paths in medicine; students are unable to comprehend the bitterly antagonistic attitudes that develop among them.

Since attitudes among the faculty can impair intraprofessional cooperation in the educational process, they become problems of prime importance. Perhaps from these problems stem greatest justification for establishment of psychology as a basic "science" in medicine. Medical education itself can to some extent bring about a degree of self-discovery in him who is educated. Except for the relatively few physicians who have had didactic analysis (psychoanalysts) it is doubtful that many clinicians or other persons attain any large degree of self-discovery until late in life, if ever. Many need not didactic analysis but forms of specialized education designed to reorganize thinking and bring about individual self-discovery.

Pertinent also to education of the physician in the alleviation of human suffering are the communications that depend upon "treaters" being able to talk to "preventers," "pure researchers" talking to "applied researchers," and pediatricians talking to internists. As in the case of certain kidney diseases, there are serious illnesses in adults, which may have been foreshadowed, possibly prevented, if detected during pediatric care of the child. While it is the way of specialists of any sort to seek their own paths in observing one or the other aspect of life's spectrum, more effective communication among specialists and generalists would bring greater benefits to patient care. In order to do this, any inherent tendencies toward egotism found among specialists or generalists must be brought into proper perspective and controlled. These tendencies are difficult to control since physicians, like most human beings, can become the center of their aims. It becomes futile for most human beings to overcome egotism entirely, and perhaps in the foreseeable future they will remain the center of their aims and seek environmental conformity to these aims. Physicians though must control this biological instinct in matters of communication and display an "altruism" in their interpersonal relationships.

When we speak of human beings generally and practitioners of the healing art particularly, we speak of a near "end product" of biological evolution who survived through egotism.* Nowa-

*William James pictured human beings as "instinctively pugnacious." Freud maintained that man's nature is such that aggression and conflict are inevitable in human relationships; he implies that at man's present state of evolution "it is an illusion to suppose that human nature can be transformed by civilization" (see Ernest Jones, *Life and Work of Sigmund Freud,* New York: Basic Books, Inc., Vol. I, 1953). On the other hand men like Ralph Waldo Emerson and in more modern times, Albert Einstein and Albert Schweitzer, believed that aggression and conflict among human beings would be overcome by civilization—it was merely a question of how soon.

days they cannot all be egotists in a biological sense and survive. This makes altruism of utmost importance in the teaching and philosophy of medicine. Altruistic seeking and accumulation of gratitude, from other members of society, have in the past been fundamental to success of well-loved family physicians and teachers in medicine. In recent medical generations this altruism has been absent both in the philosophy and teaching of medicine. It could prove a valuable, larger common goal of the healing art, as a substitute for some of its egocentric or self-priority aims. This philosophy requires a mutual seeking and accumulation of gratitude among students and teachers, full-time and part-time educators, specialists and nonspecialists, and most important, among practitioners of the healing art and the social order. Within a new and dynamic philosophy, forms of intramural hostility within the profession or toward segments of the social order would become incompatible with ultimate aims of medicine.

For lack of an altruistic philosophy in the practice of the healing art, organized medicine finds it difficult nowadays to frame ground rules for dealing with public dissatisfaction and dissident groups within its own ranks. Most lacking is a dynamic philosophy adaptable to social change in relationship to healing-art practice; i.e., in matters of freedom of choice (in contradistinction to self-determination); professional freedom of the physician in relation to the social order; and rights of patients as "free agents" in society. Much that has been propounded on these concepts by organized medicine's tired public-relation devices has shown little evidence that a new dynamic philosophy has been born—a philosophy suitable to making judicious contractural relationships with society. Too many of its responses to challenge in these relationships have been economic rather than ideologic.

When we speak of developing a new altruism in medicine there are obstructions other than human biological hostility or egotism to be considered. In the achievement of long-term goals or ultimate aims in life, practitioners and human beings generally can become entangled by the obstructive influences of too many short-term goals. While achievement of long-term goals for practitioners does not preclude the achievement of more ephemeral short-term goals, these latter goals in too great abundance can block ultimate aims.

Full devotion to professionalism of healing often precludes an epicurean life for the busy practitioner. Further, economics of hedonism may compete with other financial commitments of physicians especially those early in his training, practice, and family life. At times young physicians are tempted to place short-range ahead of the long-range goals; thus a young physician, especially if he has strong egotistic impulses, may displace partially or entirely lose sight of ultimate aims in his professional philosophy. Then the urge to accumulate gratitude becomes displaced; to earn more and more "bread" becomes a primary concern.

In the past, many loved and "successful" family practitioners were able to achieve a balance between monetary and "psychic" rewards. Nowadays, this is difficult for the majority of the profession to achieve because of economic pressures in society; thus physicians who become preoccupied with economic aims are looked upon by the public as "merchants" of medicine and surgery. Those physicians who do achieve a balance between short- and long-range goals frequently go unnoticed; still, they give great meaning and direction to their personal and professional lives. Those unsung heroes identify themselves with most of the collective aims in the social order of man; they ennoble themselves and others.

The goals and aims of physician considered above do not change the puritan or protestant ethic of work and reward, but attention has been given to the nature of rewards other than economic. To some, it may seem that noneconomic rewards would prove unattractive to those individualists who choose medicine as a career, a career requiring at times a high order of ego or egotism. This is especially true in those clinical situations where a physician must exercise individual judgment (sometimes omnipotent) as to what is best for the patient; some of these judgments are made within his purview, and are often free of interference from within or without the profession.

In opposing altruistic and worldly philosophies (economics) in the art of healing, we must consider language intimately bound to medical education. First of all, financial "investment" made in medical education, in the language of the marketplace, requires "amortization" and "capital gain" or "yield." The rate of return or yield may depend on the time and financial investment in education and training made by a particular practitioner. The more highly specialized the practitioner, the more "valuable" to himself and others he becomes each year of his life expectancy after the educational process; and he views this in relation to his original investment in time and money in the process. Thus, as a matter of urgency, short-term economic goals can easily cloud, overshadow, or block altruistic aims.

As has been mentioned, a fair return on medical education investment is forced into economic language by conditions dictated by materialistic structures and values in society. Thus individual and collective philosophies of practitioners contributing to a new general philosophy in medicine can be expected to undergo little change under these conditions. The language of investment in the healing art's educational process thus remains one expressive of devotion to profitable financial return and not one primarily of altruistic "emotional" involvement *(Agape)*.

A de-emphasis in language of investment pertaining to medical education would depend somewhat on decisions of the social order to subsidize the entire educational process. This would eliminate certain semantic barriers in the philosophy of medicine created by economic realities of society's own materialism. Favorable effects on language may already be manifest among one or two recent generations of students and practitioners who received varying amounts of subsidy in their educations.

Still remaining is an element of distrust within the social order generally and in organized medicine in particular toward the role of government in education. This could delay further evolution in the language and philosophy of medicine. There are those in medicine who fear further sociologic orientation in medical education under the aegis of government. They feel this may disturb homeostatic equilibrium within the organized profession. Meanwhile authoritarian planning in government as a rule goes on and anticipates socioeconomic problems in delivery of medical care well in advance of the medical profession's leadership; so the security or homeostasis of organized medicine and its leadership is under continuing threat of dynamic social planning and change.

There are other obstructions to a philosophy of altruism in the practice of the healing art. These stem from semantic difficulties inherent in the use by the profession of words "prerogative" and "privilege."* Physicians are granted privileges of rendering medical services under law; some may feel only those having attained an educational degree to practice this privilege should plan for the delivery of these services. Here professional *privilege* is confused with *prerogative* of social planning inherent in most forms of government. Reasoning often expressed here is that social planners being unable to treat the sick *ergo* are unable to plan for the delivery of such services to human beings. Attempt at "partnership" with the social order in planning delivery of medical care is still considered by some, in organized medicine, as fallacious "reasoning." In its nostalgic myopia, organized medicine still cites a glorious history of accomplishments in healing throughout the centuries without aid of authoritarian or polity planning. In all such *apologias,* realities of problems created by medicine's technical advancements are overlooked; these realities, by their very nature, necessitate planning by the polity in an evolving social order.

Even if major socioeconomic obstacles to a new altruism in the philosophy of medicine can be modified or eliminated and most practitioners as individuals could relate to this altruism from the time of early training, an unfinished task would remain. This task would lie in the field of the psychological education of physicians.

Nowadays, a large segment of our society is knowledgeable, through formal or informal education, in matters involving psychological data or principles of human behavior. This important

---

*Members of the medical profession at times equate "privileges," "rights," and "prerogatives" *generally* with individual freedom in personal action in the attainment of goals for themselves and patients.

aspect of knowledge, until recently, received little recognition in premedical or medical education as a prerequisite of training in the understanding of "persons" with or without mental illnesses. In addition to its importance as a stimulus to early self-discovery among students of medicine, study of psychology appears basic to understanding the practice of medicine in the way that anatomy and physiology are considered basic "sciences." Only a few medical schools today recognize this and have moved in this direction in design of curricula.

In the fruition of a new dynamic philosophy in medicine, it is important for the physician to know himself (physician know thyself); also to step outside of himself, in evaluating reactions to other human beings and clinical events and his own limitations. He practices an art within areas of intuition connected with powers of judgment in which he must know himself well—his total life situation, emotions, prejudices, neuroticisms. When symbolic or verbal language of clinical situations arise, his intuitive sense must tell him all is not well. He must know his deficiencies and when necessary humbly pursue help from others. If in difficult clinical situations a physician does not know "who he is," his image becomes even more disorganized in the minds of patients, their families, and colleagues especially when clinical situations deteriorate. The education of practitioners toward this degree of self-discovery is closely related to future tasks of medicine and to dynamic changes in health needs within the social order.

Student selection and medical education orientated along the paths of psychological as well as in social sciences and humanities would diminish many obstacles to the acceptance of a philosophy of altruism *(Agape)* in the healing art. Whether as a result we could expect the bulk of practitioners to at first admit altruism as an ultimate aim, or making patients or others in society grateful, is dubious. Practitioners who may sacrifice a great deal of their private lives for practices would deny accumulation of gratitude as a goal or motivation. They may, in fact, express an element of surprise that what they may consider a selfish, even naive motive could influence professional efforts in healing the sick. Considered more socially acceptable and less selfish to them are reasons of science for science's sake, art for art's sake, service to others, challenge of the task, economic rewards, prestige, and approval. All of these on scrutiny become no less selfish in motivation than inspiration of gratitude among others. All such reasons upon close examination are those subconsciously planned to earn gratitude or approval from others. Even an anonymous saint of untold or unsung virtues and sacrifices in the end may wish approval, albeit from a divine rather than human source.

To consider fully a philosophy of medicine based on altruism, we must give special attention to the nature of "benefits" applicable to behavior of human beings in relation to what they believe to be their self- or best interests. Most human beings ask and seek proof that these interests are being served.* Receptiveness to ministrations or directives of a physician, or others in a society, is based on expectations of either positive benefits or of the losses that will be prevented by the relationship.

Prevention, removal, or diminution of threat of imminent loss is at times as important as positive gain in the workings of human relationships. It is within this more negative context that most of the healing art (anticipatory and curative medicine) is practiced. Illness is considered by most human beings as an alienating loss.

It is through either prevention or modification of illness in a manner favorable to the sick individual that services of physicians become benefits to individuals. Thus any consideration of altruism (based on accumulation of gratitude) is inseparable from consideration of the nature and kinds of benefits involved in the patient-physician relationship. Furthermore, we can postulate that the true measure of *caritas* in a practitioner of the healing art is his ability and willingness to bring benefits to others.

When speaking of bringing benefits to individual patients we speak not only of the patient's self-priorities but the interests of

---

*The pessimistic and often despairing philosophy of Schopenhauer (*The World As Will And Idea*) treats this as a matter of cynical pessimism rather than altruistic optimism in human relationships.

his family, friends, relatives, or any person whose welfare he may have at heart. Thus what physicians often look on as an exclusively individual ethical focus in relationships is really multiphasic. Choices of "right" benefits applicable to an individual necessarily involve multiphasic analysis of good- and poor-quality actions not only in relationship to the individual but to a community ethical focus. Facility in translating good- and poor-quality actions into benefits and losses, with multiphasic considerations, can be only partially based on strictly medical technical skill. A greater degree may depend upon the physician's broad nonmedical awareness of the patient as a member of the social order and oftentimes on factors beyond the purview of medical practice.

The common notion that the self-interest of the patient is totally defined by his physiological integrity often proves erroneous. As complications of purely medical or surgical technical judgments, physicians also must decide whether certain benefits brought to the patient by a medical or surgical procedure outweigh losses to the patient—not only economic but those in body comfort, temporary or permanent, which may be expected by physicians as concomitant or necessary evils of medical and surgical procedures. These decisions are the most complex form of multiphasic analysis in benefits and losses. They occur frequently after the problems in technical judgment are resolved. Then multiphasic analysis proceeds from the individual to the community ethical focus, including family, friends, and relatives.

Represented schematically are some of the complexities in determination of right benefits that the practitioner must choose for a patient in relationship to factors in the total life situation of the patient.

As a benefit of surgery, one could expect relief from pain, improvement in organic health of the patient. Except in rare cases of persons with emotional dependency on symptoms, successful surgery would decrease symptoms and even effect an improved emotional status in the individual. Possible losses to the patient would be those physiological and symptomatic changes in the gastrointestinal tract as a result of surgery (dumping syndrome). Economic losses to the patient over and above in-

Should Patient Have Partial Gastrectomy?				
	YES—Surgery		NO—Continue Medication or Conservative ℞	
	Benefits	Losses	Benefits	Losses
1. Patient	+ + +	- -	+	- - - -
2. Physician	+ + +	?	+ +	- -
3. Family	+ + +	?	?	?
4. Community	+ +		+ +	
5. Employer	+ +	- - -		- - - -

demnification insurance for hospital and medical care or possible loss of wages also are considerations.

A family may benefit from the patient's surgery in that the patient functions organically as a more effective father or husband, able to report more regularly to his job. There is the element of mortality risk in surgery, depending on the preoperative clinical picture; and the family could sustain a great loss.

On either side of the affirmative and negative decision, the physician could sustain a personal loss in serenity provoked by normal anxiety.* This would be concomitant with the rigorousness of the medical technical decision making and the weighing of risk factors with other factors in the patient's total life situation. Unless the physician does the major surgery himself economic

*More common day to day occurrences in medical practice are decisions made with regard to use of potent medications where there is calculated risk of side effects of drugs or antibiotics; these must be weighed in light of proven effectiveness of the medication in particular types of diseases. Good intentions and enthusiasm for drugs often do patients more harm than good. There are many medications being used today of doubtful efficiency but of conclusively proven toxicity. Here the art of medicine frequently supersedes the science of medicine. Other examples are those decisions that must be made daily by physicians as to whether patients should remain in intensive care units "one more day"; these decisions must be weighed in light of patient condition, the need of other patients in the hospital, and the exorbitant expense to patients connected with use of intensive care units.

considerations in benefits to himself would be negligible in the decision. Regardless of who performs the surgery, he can lose patient and family gratitude should the multiphasic analysis he did of the situation prove too limited in scope. What was thought to be a major benefit may be considered by the patient a loss. Extreme constriction in his analysis could make the physician culpable and censurable.

If we postulate the economic "health" of a community to be affected by the health status of those living in that community, successful surgery in the individual patient then would be a benefit to the community. If as a result of surgery the individual becomes physically or emotionally handicapped the community could sustain an economic loss, either in welfare payments or in public payment for continuing medical and hospital expense.

While most employers' interest in an employee's illness may be at first humanitarian, often in cases of prolonged illness the employers' concern becomes "ledgerized" with economic considerations at times outweighing humanitarian ones. This is especially true of employers who on an unindemnified basis (out of pocket) contribute to sick leave "benefits." Should the employee survive successful surgery and the employer persevere in humanitarianism, the employer can benefit by return to work of an individual who is in better health, able to perform his work regularly and with greater ease. Should the employee not survive surgery, the economic loss to the employer is mainly in terms of losing a human being valuable to the work force. In some instances a loss is sustained by life insurance companies on the actuarial basis of calculating group life insurance plans.

In the schematic presentation of multiphasic analysis an activist "yes" decision was represented. More difficult decisions for the practitioners are those of nonsurgical intervention ("no" decision). Here, the multiphasic analysis of benefits and losses presents to the physician choices in losses to the patient so as to achieve what he or the patient may consider one or two important benefits of nonintervention. For example, if there already is a serious illness problem in the home of the patient or a serious problem at work, the most important benefit to the patient may be to remain ambulatory in order to attend work or assist some sick member of his family. His family or employer thus may benefit even though the patient himself could sustain losses in the form of serious complications of his illness. Complications could become serious enough over a period of delay making him a poor surgical risk. Increasing disability could affect his relationship with the employer to the extent that eventually he and his family could become indigent or public "charges" in the community. What the physician can accomplish for him in the way of treatment may be less in the future than the present. The success of the physician in an activist role may diminish in proportion to time lapse in postponement of surgery. Quantitative losses exceed benefits in the decision "not to operate." However, to the patient there is *the one benefit* already mentioned that he *believes* to be qualitatively more important to his own best interests at work and to those of his family. He believes *the one benefit* outweighs quantitative preponderance of losses.

The choice of the right decision (good-quality action) for the patient, potentially a godlike one, can go beyond the individual ethical focus and often is more than a matter of pure medical or surgical judgment. Once a judgment or choice is made this must be translated into language of benefits so the patient will understand and more important *believe* that the choice produces *the benefit* he feels is to his own and the interests of others dear to him.

True measure of a physician within the *caritas* concept becomes then not only a matter of ability and willingness to bring benefits to patients but to earn gratitude, the ability to convince or make patients believe particular benefits to be in their *best* interests. It is within the context of patient belief that the language of present-day medicine becomes deficient in relationship to its progress.

If, cybernetically, the schema of multiphasic analysis in benefit and loss could be programmed, the value judgments made in individual cases involving the physician-patient relationship would present serious difficulties. These difficulties would be apparent in the selection in an individual case of the right benefits in relationship to concomitant or nonconcomitant losses. More difficult would be the task of making the patient *believe* in *the right benefit* chosen through computer programming.

To complicate such programming are a host of governing influences (instinctive and intellectual) that determine right benefits for particular individuals seeking medical care. These are influenced by needs of the individual beyond physiological integrity, beyond food, clothing, and shelter; they encompass emotional security, social-order identity, belonging, recognition, and respect as an individual. These needs all enter into the patient-physician relationships and become of paramount importance in efforts to obtain favorable attention of patients in the relationships. Without them attempts in gaining a favorable listening process so benefits and losses can be reasoned and verbalized often become futile.

The philosophy of benefit and loss in human motivation is complicated by those in the minority (some are neurotic) who do not believe or act in terms of appreciation of benefits or losses. The majority of people believe and act according to benefits they appreciate as being important to their short-term goals or ultimate aims. Whether they listen, in order to believe, becomes another matter, which involves the problem of language usage generally in gaining favorable attention of patients or other persons so they may listen to benefits.

Appeals by practitioners to patients or families to listen to benefits of decision making involve at times emotion movers based on reason coming from within the practitioner. These must be presented in specific and believable language and with sincerity and *caritas*. The degree practitioners are able to convince patients or their families of their sincerity in use of emotion movers may determine the degree of acceptance and gratitude. True *caritas* based on reason allows no room for quackery in mood or manner at bedsides.

The word "sincerity" though both an object and subject noun has true meaning only in relation to internal qualities of human motivation and action. Nor can it be a mask worn according to particular clinical situations. It comes from within the physician and is based on reason, humility, *Agape*, and the courage of his convictions. Human beings value and appreciate highly this quality in physicians. Sincere (without wax) interest on the part of the physician, in itself, is a therapeutic modality, which in the art of medicine can cause improvement in patients even in the most serious and disabling forms of disease.

We must consider further the quality of humility in the philosophy of medicine as to whether it is in conflict with the practitioner's pride in accomplishment. A great part of the cultural milieu today is affected by the technological climate we live in. Humility has become unpopular and considered undesirable by some in society who respond to challenges of technology. A world precocious in technology at times makes *impossible* or *incredible* old-fashioned, even obsolete, words. One-upmanship in all forms of technology—medical, surgical, and in other fields of human endeavor—has become obsessional among many responding to present-day technological challenges. This is evidenced by the consternation, even shame, suffered by individuals, groups, cultures, and nations when others surpass their technological efforts, be these in medicine, surgery, chemistry, physics, or space technology. With this momentum operative within societies, often the challenge of long-term basic problems of people do not stimulate proportionate responses in society. Often, diseases such as malaria, diphtheria, or cholera thought extinct by many, become rampant in parts of the world at the same time that a zenith is reached in space technology. New microcosms and worlds are discovered, leaving the problems of the old unsolved in part or whole.

Heretofore philosophers employed the concept of truth as something dependent upon facts largely beyond human control. In this manner they inculcated the necessary element of humility into serious thinking in science and art. This check upon pride has been removed and scientific investigators have succumbed to thinking that man's present powers are sufficient for any task in the universe. For those in medicine to succumb to this notion denudes them of necessary equanimity.

With mankind's ever-extending reach to grasp the impossible and the incredible, can a reasonable value judgment be made on the virtue of humility as a necessary part of the philosophy of medicine? Further, as a quality of action in thought or deed, does it have relevance to the practitioner's ability or willingness to bring benefits to patients or communities? Benefits related not only to his immediate material self-interests but to his greater ultimate aims? Would a sense of genuine or sincere humility affect favorably or unfavorably the carrying out of his responsibilities? These at times approach spheres of omnipotence in action and make him subject to warranty as a deity rather than as a fallible human being.

There is also the question of evolutionary forces. What has been discovered of such powers certainly have not been inventions of man but the partial or full discovery by man of their workings. In considering the causality of these workings man may or may not need a hypothesis even though one would be extremely useful, especially if he seeks points of reference outside his own material existence. In discussing the powers affecting the intricate order of things, the word "nature" is difficult to avoid in reference to causality, even though semantically it erroneously implies that nature as a subject of a transitive verb is acting upon objects as evolving animate and inanimate orders. Causality, though its manifestation be considered "accidental," continues to be the nameless entity of "doer," recognized but deleted in the deliberations of many scientific groups in the name of objectivity.

That such objectivity is easily or fully attained may be a brash assumption even among most eminent of medical scientists. The limits to such objectivity most difficult to overcome are those unseen, since we are not able to examine our own limits of "rationality," only the limits of its functions or manifestations (pragmatic). What we objectively call instinct, intellect, mind, central nervous system really become presumptions in a metaphysical, ontological, and semantic sense.

Philosophers and physicists (Bergson, Einstein) readily have given credence to limits of objectivity when striving to learn truth about the world through techniques of observation and analysis. Some in the physical, biological, and health sciences, who for lack of humility or objective self-appraisal, persist in recognizing no such limits. Most as a matter of habit use language within some practical frame of reference. This language tends to be saturated from childhood with habits and concepts strongly bound to carry-over and new frames of reference. Frequently medical and other types of scientists attempt to overcome this by using greater specificity or precision in language. Even then word usages may continue to reflect long-established preconceptions. They have been looking and speaking of a world through personal frames of reality too long to completely transcend old thought or language patterns. They recognize no barriers to their knowledge other than the time required to superimpose on the old additional practical frames of reference. Some are prone to discover an already existing but heretofore unknown natural force and call it their own invention. If it can be copied it becomes their "creation." Allowed a few physical biochemical or biological postulates, some will on paper design an evolving biopsychosocial order in a universe of their own making.

Limitations in objective powers of observation place the human body in the perspective of a special type of machine responding in a practical and an abstract sense to other types of machines in its environment. That its own responses are limited is evidenced by the many influences in its external or internal environments to which it fails to respond, at least immediately. For instance, human beings ordinarily are not sensitive to radio waves unless these are converted into electrical impulses and sound.

To the extent that the human being is able to discover more and more of unknown influences, he becomes increasingly a greater witness to his own creative powers but also his own evolution within. Many of the ultimate realities of the universe and our existence may be quite beyond reach of biological and other sciences in the present stage of the human evolutionary process, a stage where many barriers to comprehension exist in the human mind. Older and more learned physicians admit that these barriers exist readily; the less learned, young and old, reluctantly.

As long as an ethos and knowledgeable "truth" remain desirable goals in an evolving social order, a sense of humility, be it termed self-discovery or honest self-appraisal, both in success and failure, would seem to have relevance to medicine's philosophy as an essential attribute among physicians. As a corollary it would also appear under our present state of knowledge that there may be things that are impossible or incredible within mortal frames of reference but possible or credible within points of reference of unknown or unrecognized powers in the evolutionary scheme of things in the animate and inanimate world. Historically as man discovered the unknown or unrecognized he changed the genesis of his philosophy through reevaluation of himself in relation to new discovery (Copernican Thought Revolution).*

Those, especially medical educators, concerned with the precarious position of the healing art, its confusion and loss of direction, propose new sets of values in medical education as necessary to development of new self-concepts among physicians. Medical educators would accomplish this in revising curricular content and teaching methods so that the span of learning and competence of practitioners would, in a dynamic sense, be relevant to the health needs of the people. They propose not only to increase medical school admissions but to encourage a greater diversity in the ethnic, geographic, and economic backgrounds and awarenesses among the applying students. Curricula would be individualized to fit students' achievement ability, educational background, and career goal-orientation. Such proposals mentioned comprise a practical supply and demand response to the challenge for new values but contain bright overtones of hope and promise for the future of medicine in an expanded awareness.

Most significant among the responses of medical educators to the challenges for a new value system would be emphasis on responsibility not only for medical research achievement but research on how these achievements can be best delivered to

*One of the four great "shocks" towards pride or ego, along with the Darwinian and Freudian *Theories;* it displaced man from center of universe. Darwin displaced him from unique position in Animal World; Freud postulated that man was not master of his own mind. The new discoveries in space may find man a "prisoner" of earth.

people. This would include those communities distant from the vertical mounds of teaching and research institutions.

These responses represent the results of "institutional" self-appraisals in relation to changes in the value system in the philosophy of medicine. Do they apply to values fundamental to the philosophy among the individual human beings who enter medical schools as students? We might assume that the established values among most of these individuals are solid, that the students are committed to *caritas, equalitas,* and *fraternitas.* Admittedly, some may have forgotten these values but could be easily reminded of them. Both assumptions may overlook an *existential crisis* problem for those in the social order who have to varying degrees lost the capacity or power to affirm any values, no matter how important their content may appear.

In addition to already discussed factors in motivation among those who seek a career in medicine we find value preferences often characteristic of religious and ethnic groups. Today in a good percentage we still find *homo economicus* who emphasize the primary importance of good income and prestige and the secondary importance of close identifying relationships with the social order and contribution to human knowledge. Some under-play economic and prestigious motivations and emphasize values related to seeking objective certainty in knowledge. There are many whose value profiles do not match but approach the two aforementioned characteristics; others seek mainly independent action spheres in a medical career. Some correlations can also be seen between religiosity and personality characteristics of authoritarianism and Machiavellianism. Those identified with the former tend to select general practice and reject internal medicine, psychiatry, teaching, and research; those with the latter reject general practice and may overselect psychiatry and research.

When value profiles such as mentioned exist, there can be no assurance that the birth of a new philosophy in medicine will result from a strictly institutional reappraisal of its values—from changing the content and methods of medical education. Medical school students, seeking paths of progress toward individual goals, could contribute to a new philosophy if schooled in development of inner capacities to affirm, experience, and most important accept internally values *out of the heart* where real ethical issues of life dwell; i.e., love or caring, equality, and brotherhood. There would be less need for external ethical rules (Thou shalt not) in the profession if external actions of the practitioner became one with these inner issues and motives. Value preferences based on this concept would be useful to the physician's ultimate aim in gaining gratitude among his fellow man. It may bind him more securely to an economy of human values in his labors among the afflicted.

What manner of human being can be expected to perform best within the philosophy of medicine discussed? The paradox is that the young are of optimum age for the learning process in medicine but often not old or wise enough for total commitment tc social order or to the healing art. To perform best within the philosophy would require emergence from egocentricity in order to take active, mature, sincere interest in the needs of others. The physician must mature more rapidly than his fellow men; some never do. In any event, since most human beings mature and shed many egocentric propensities, it would appear that barriers to older persons in the study of medicine would seem artificial and perhaps not in the best interests of the profession. It requires an inordinate amount of time, simply because of his age, for the average young physician to establish mature relationships with his patients and with life generally; and this may impair greatly the development of his potentialities.

Many of those who enter the study of medicine later in life become successful practitioners within the context of the philosophy discussed. Whether these individuals come from the ranks of laicized clergy, missionary laymen, law, or from biological and physical sciences, they often bring a philosophy and maturity committing them to greater accomplishment and involvement in the solution of problems in the psychosocial order. They bring with them a language of awareness that is less constricted than among most of those whose initial vocation is the study and practice of medicine. Many have learned to speak in terms of moral decisions and responsibilities that affect others in society besides themselves, responsibilities not only to their immediate profession but to the community, the nation, and the world. Their language is derived from a sense of well-being and security in accomplishing what they consider good for their patients and society in general. Much of the success in their interpersonal relationships depends upon emotional maturity, a *sine qua non* in the practice of the healing art.

Since we must continue to train young persons for careers in medicine we must tackle the realities of effecting the greatest possible concentricity of motivations and value preferences within the philosophy of medicine. Those who visualize batteries of psychological or other tests* effecting this concentricity must realize that even if we could with accuracy identify *homo caritas* among *homo economicus, homo australopithecus,* or *homo omnipotensis,* it would only be the beginning of the solution. Like in all psychological testing, godlike decisions remain as to whether some types should be educated "into" and others "outside" the profession. It is conceivable that a partial solution would be paths of progress in lifelong education, a guidance aimed at self-discovery among students monitored by teachers responsible for their education and later guidance by senior colleagues in practice. As indicated this would be a lifelong process since the philosophy of medicine as well as its techniques would remain dynamic and value preferences of individuals would be subject to change. As new challenges require new responses it is conceivable we may need in medicine in addition to *homo caritas* some, hopefully not many, types** other than those whose ultimate aim is the accumulation of gratitude among men. Along these paths of lifelong education and guidance the language of the healing art in its dialogue with the social order would be subject

*Applications and indices (Q.P.I.) used in selective process have been standardized for all medical schools in the United States; college performance (academic and in the sciences) is heavily weighted in selection.

**Later we will consider the need for these types of practitioners should the polity give wholesale sanction to "exterminative medicine" in population control.

to the dynamics of change in the goals and ultimate aims of the profession so as to be at one with its inner motives.

In envisioning any plan of teaching that would provide comprehensive systems of guidance and counseling, medical educators could no longer be available for predominantly administrative duties. Equality and brotherhood among students and faculty would necessarily prevail in the learning process; teachers would find little time for duties other than those requiring active and personal involvement with the student body.* Continuation of this process after graduation would require changes not only in the size, character, and communications of various segments of organized medicine but in preoccupations, from external to the internal affairs of its members. In this manner the language of organized medicine would become less external, economic, exploitative and more in keeping with the inward motives or attitudes of *caritas*, *equalitas*, and *fraternitas*.

What preprofessional educational awareness would be relevant to a new dynamic philosophy of medicine? Certainly in addition to a thorough knowledge of his own language and culture and a reasonable knowledge of the language and cultures of others, the student will need an increasing amount of integrative skill not necessarily related to biological or physical sciences. Before using patients as a "text" in the development of integrative skill, the pursuit in preprofessional years of those humanities that teach basic scales, chords, and triads in the polyphonic composition of human relationships would seem relevant. Though by orientation in scientific methods in his pre-professional schooling he may have developed a remarkable capacity to collect exhaustive series of facts, his powers of synthesis and integrative skill may fail him in the appraisal of the *total* patient situation unless he has skills derived from the humanities, giving him insight into language, personality, economics, sociology. In addition, integrative skill so derived along with knowledge of disease mechanisms and dynamics allows for judicious assignment of priorities in total clinical evaluation and management of the patient. There is little

*Close human relationship of "master" and "apprentice."

time during or after medical school training for the indoctrination of integrative skill.

Medicine today represents within itself a remarkable synthesis of science and art; it has become increasingly apparent that the same synthesis is crucial to preprofessional education, to preparing those who must learn later the comprehensive integration of individual patients. Without knowledge or skill in the integrative process physicians lose the true art of medicine. Successful synthesis of this sort, whether it be in medicine, theoretical physics, writing, painting, sculpture, or music, requires a broad basis of awareness.

In this discussion it is important to remember that the social order generally must produce types of individuals deemed suitable or unsuitable to any philosophy of medicine. The evolution of the healing art therefore becomes intimately bound to the general evolutionary phenomenon of man, particularly in its ethical or spiritual and social directions. That man has at least a partial choice in the latter seems evident by directional choices in the field of technology already made. There is good reason to believe that the evolutionary path of man ahead is more and more toward the collective good of the psychosocial order, even though from time to time there are derailments. We would expect with this momentum that the social order would produce more and more human beings suitable to its needs in medicine and other fields and more and more individuals whose attributes are compatible with its goals. The question here is what degree of alacrity will dominant majorities guiding the future of the healing art display in recognizing or identifying those members of society best suited to a new philosophy.

Perhaps at this stage man is so taken up by new discoveries in science that he is in the serious predicament of not having time or energy to devote to philosophical implications of discovery. Long time lags continue to occur between advancements in medicine and fulfillment of expectations relating to these advancements, since at present man's social evolution becomes temporarily sidetracked by his preoccupation with scientific analysis. To complicate matters the human race has made the words *education* and *intelligence* synonymous to a large degree, forgetting that education becomes only a catalyst to capability factors inherent in intelligence. For the physician, in his education and philosophy, it appears at present that acceptance of the *Agape** quotient is equal in importance to his acceptance of the intelligence or knowledge quotient. Further, regardless of whether one believes or not that altruism belongs to the nature of man, its acceptance may no longer be a matter of choice for the physician or all other human beings.

*Here we employ the word *agape* as a "conscious acceptance and thorough *relatedness* to all other human beings," described by J. Samuel Bois. See *Explorations in Awareness,* J. Samuel Bois, New York: Harper & Row, 1957.

Alvey, C. R. "Family Physician as Educator." *JAMA,* 177:763-764 (Sept.) 1961.

Blanton, Smiley. *Love or Perish.* New York: Simon and Schuster, 1956.

Bronowski, J. *Science and Human Values.* New York: Julian Messner, Inc., 1956.

Califano, Joseph, H. *The Student Revolution.* New York: W. W. Norton & Co., 1969.

Castiglioni, A. *History of Medicine.* New York: Alfred A. Knopf, 1941.

Clark, W. E. Le Gros. *History of the Primates.* Chicago: The University of Chicago Press, 1961.

Cooper, John A. D. "Expanding Dimensions of Medicine." *JAMA*, Vol. 185, No. 5 (Aug. 3), 1963.

Coye, R. D., Itausen M. F. "The Doctors Assistant," *Journal Amer. Med. Association,* Vol. 204, No. 4 (July 28, 1969).

de Chardin, Teilhard. *The Phenomenon of Man.* New York and Evanston: Harper & Row, 1961.

Deuschle, Kurt W. "Training Physicians for Family Medicine." *JAMA,* Vol. 181, No. 5 (Aug. 4), 1962.

Eiseley, Loren. *The Immense Journey.* New York: Random House Inc., 1962.

Ellis, H. "Place of Anthropology in Medical Education." *Lancet,* 2:365-366, 1892.

Freud, Sigmund. "Beyond the Pleasure Principle."

Harvey, S. C. "Objectives of Medical Education." *Yale .J. Biol. Med.,* 13:847-862, 1941.

Hunt, Andrew D., Jr. "Medical Schools and Health Care Research." *Arch. Environmental Health,* Vol. 18 (Feb.), 1969.

Hunt, William A. "Professional Interaction Between Psychology and Medicine." *Pre-Med,* 2:18-24, 1962.

Jonas, Adolph D. "The Case for Theoretical Medicine." *JAMA,* Vol. 184, No. 13 (June 29), 1963.

Jones, Ernest. *The Life and Works of Sigmund Freud.* Vol. I. New York: Basic Books, 1959.

Kepler, Milton O. "Can the Art of Medicine Survive?" *Medical Annals District of Columbia,* May, 1967.

Kruse, H.D. "Medical Education, Medical Practice and Medical Care." *Bull. N. Y. Acad. Med.,* 73:311-341 (May), 1961.

Magoun, H. W.; Darling, Louise; and Prost, J. *The Evolution of Man's Brain.* New York: Josiah Macy, Jr. Foundation, 1960.

McKittrick, Leland. "Valuable Goals for the Medical School." *JAMA,* Vol. 185, No. 2. (July 13), 1963.

Montague, Ashley. "Anthropology and Medical Education." *JAMA,* Vol. 183, No. 7 (Feb. 16), 1963.

Montague, Ashley. *On Being Human*. New York: Henry Schuman, 1951.

Oppenheimer, O. "Science and the Human Community" in *Issues in University Education*, Charles Frankel (ed.). New York: Harper and Brothers, 1959, pp. 48-62.

Pequinot, H. "Scientific and Social Aspects of Medicine." *Impact* (Unesco), 51:203-259, 1954.

Psychology and the Problems of Society. Korten, Francis F.; Cook, Stuart W.; Lacey, John J. (eds). Washington D.C.: The American Psychological Assoc., 1970.

Randall, O. A. "The Essential Partnership of Medicine and Social Work." *Geriatrics*, 5:46 (Jan. to Feb.), 1950.

Reichart, K. "Some Aspects of the Relationship Between Private Physicians and Social Agencies." Unpublished doctorate thesis, University of Minnesota, 1955.

Richardson, H. B. *Patients Have Families*. The Commonwealth Fund, New York, 1945.

Richmond, Julius, B. *Currents in American Medicine—A Developmental View of Medical Care and Education*. Cambridge, Mass.: Harvard University Press, 1969.

Robbins, Paul R.; Myersburg, Norman. "A Medical Student's Awareness, Psychologic Factors—An Exploratory Study." *Medical Annals*. Dist. of Columbia. Vol. 38, No. 6 (June), 1969.

Roberts, C. "Anthropology for Medical Students." *Lancet*, 2:456-457, 1892.

Rogers, David E. "A Dean's List of Proposals." *Med. Opinion & Reviews,* (Oct.) 1969.

Rutstein, D. D. "Physicians for Americans, Two New Medical Curricula, New Proposal." *Lancet*, 1:498-501 (March), 1961.

Seyle, Hans. *The Stress of Life,* Book V. New York-Toronto-London: McGraw-Hill Book Co. Inc.

Simmons, L. W., and Wolff, H. G. *Social Science in Medicine*. New York: Russell Sage Foundation, 1954.

Simpson, G. G. *The Meaning of Evolution*. New Haven: Yale University Press, 1949.

Sorokin, Pitrim (ed.). *Explorations in Altruistic Love and Behaviour*. Boston: The Beacon Press, 1950.

Travis, B. B. "Social Considerations in Patient Management," *Public Health Reports*, 70:1155 (Dec.), 1955.

Vallbona, C. "The Usefulness of Computers in the Management of the Chronically Ill and Disabled." Birmingham, Alabama: *Southern Medical Bulletin*. Vol. 57, No. 3 (Sept.), 1969.

Wagner, Robert R. "Basic Medical Sciences, Revolution in Biology and Future of Medical Education." *Yale J. Biol. Med.*, 35:1-11, 1962.

Weiner, Norbert. *The Human Use of Human Beings*. New York: Doubleday, 1954.

Wilson, J. Walter. "Sciences of New Importance to Medicine." *JAMA*, Vol. 185, No. 5. (Aug. 3) 1963.

Wilson, W. F.; Templeton, A., Turrer, A. H., and Ledwick, G. S. "The Computer Analysis and Prognosis of Gastric Ulcers," *Radiology* 85:1064, 1965.

Wood, W. B., Jr. *From Miasmas to Molecules*. New York: Columbia University Press, 1961.

CHAPTER IV

The Verbal World in the Organization and Governing of Medical Research

The organization and government of scientific research epitomizes the great proportion of human energy devoted to the pursuit of truth. If we examine the healing art and its philosophy in its broad aspects, we must give thought to directional forces at work in its research.

In organization, all research programs become literally the "crash" variety, in proportion to time lag between analysis and discovery phase and period of retrospection required to formulate philosophical implications. In the healing art, as previously indicated, the amount of energy devoted to the study of disease has not been matched by amounts of research devoted to how newly discovered truths best serve individual patients in the overall improvement of medical care.

Tracing historically the development of research, it becomes apparent that while born out of internal exuberance and curiosity of idle dreamers, modern research has taken on materialistic trappings and social status of a successful industry. As its language became more economic in character, the more its efforts became subordinated to discovery and progress in industrial and armament technology. The smaller proportion of human energy and revenue devoted to pure basic research in pursuit of truth in biological, physical, or social sciences also has engendered a language of economics.*

*Academic leaders in medical circles today speak a language indistinguishable from that of stock-market analysts. For instance, they refer to curtailment of funds in present-day research as a needed "market correction" and hope for new periods of healthy growth. In the same vein, "If the crunch is sufficiently hard, it will compel clear thinking, reassessment, and discriminating choice." They add, "There was bound to be some maldistribution of resources (funded research projects) under conditions of 'easy money,' and a 'shake out' will be good."

Historically man has been reluctant to look at himself in pursuit of truth, preferring to look at things around him. He has found self-confrontation inescapable in the alpha to the present state of his evolution. Man has had to confront himself again and again, to search for truth about himself—a truth necessary to his understanding the ultimate reality of things, such as energy, he discovered in the physical order of the universe. The knowledge obtained about stars and planets affected his philosophy (Copernican revolution in thought).

Judging by his technological discoveries man will find research about himself as time consuming and essential as that expended in the discovery and research of things outside of himself. This is especially true in regard to those discoveries that pose a threat to his reaching a higher stage of evolution. A high order of priority in the future must be given to care and improvement of the human machine. If mankind's thinking is to continue to evolve it must continue to be safely housed in a structure capable of withstanding stress placed upon it by the growth of the "mind." To date the wear and tear on the human machine caused by the awakening of the mind to new discovery has been severe.

So far, man has allowed a seemingly random development in evolution of his mind and body by natural selective processes within humanity's common gene pool. This is being challenged by an important segment of medical researchists, namely the biogeneticists. In the language of eugenics and genetics the word "nature" either as a subject or object becomes involved in, "Who knows best, man or what could be a mirage called "nature"; i.e., a supposedly infallible entity representing the forces of man's external and internal environments.

Modern man believes at this point that he can guide his future evolution through organization of his research. This implies that heretofore his role has been a passive one and he now wishes an active one by virtue of his accomplishments. He is no longer content to witness his own evolution but wishes to cause it. He may find that even prior to his mastery of scientific analysis and discovery that he already has played a principal role as a "natural" force at work in his own evolution.

With discovery of Mendelian principles in inherited characteristics, man became engrossed in scientific analysis of the significance of imprints in his genetic chemistry. He later proceeded to
analyze chemical codes of inheritance, discovered their chemical
structure, and is now busily engaged in further analysis of genetic
material. This brings him close to the day when he may tinker
with the common gene pool of humanity.

Since research in genetics plays an important part in understanding certain disease mechanisms, it must be mentioned in relation to the philosophy of medicine. First however we must consider some semantic problems inherent in terms, definitions, and
awareness in this field.

Semantic difficulties confronted in medical research are inherent in methodology of data collecting and observations where data
on laboratory animals are transposed or extrapolated to fit human
models. The microbiologists, geneticists, or biochemists may speak
different languages depending on whether they have utilized in
experimental methods *Drosophila* (fruit flies,) hamsters, mice,
monkeys, or donkeys. Semantic difficulties encountered are similar
to those occurring when astrophysicists speak to industrialists in
the garment business.

There is a gulf in language between researchists doing microbial
or laboratory animal genetics and those doing human genetics.
This becomes understandable when we consider the awareness
of those performing planned experiments on microbes and animals, in contrast to those human geneticists mainly concerned
with studying experiments on human beings who have evolved
without "experimental" programming. Within separate worlds of
events, investigators dealing with rats and mice may speak of
human world population problems in terms of sigmoid growth
curves and cessation of breeding due to crowded animal cages.
Investigators in the field of human genetics have a different awareness, namely that of man, who though rational in thought frequently is irrational in action. Discussion between these researchists, let us say, on quantitative feeding or social problems of rapid
population growth could become taut with semantic tensions, due
to a lack of language congruity.

Language impediments occur also in the dialogue of those in animal experimentation and those making human observation studies in metabolism, carcinogenecity, or ovulation. In their pre-occupations, investigators may acquire a great deal of knowledge and reverence toward animal experimental models or the physiology of particular organs. Nephrologists working with kidneys may proclaim in jest the comparative superiority of the kidney to the physiologists doing research on lungs. Biologists working with sea turtles may point with pride to the superiority of this animal to the human being by virtue of the animal's ability (by use of a coelomic cavity) to regulate acid base balances in metabolizing sugar under anaerobic (without oxygen) conditions. Investigators studying mechanisms of carbon dioxide tensions and carbonate buffering processes develop an awareness of the whole of evolution of man in terms of the "evolution" of these processes in organisms.

Those studying the Ciracidan rhythms of sea urchins and other animals often think in terms of biological rather than mechanical or atomic clocks and may have semantic difficulties with those who work mainly in the physical sciences. Difficulty in interdisciplinary language lies in fragmentation of totality in organisms, with extreme specializations of interest affecting language. Difficulties are compounded by the confusion of titles and disciplines in research where in close quarters there is an overlapping of skills and interests among investigators working in separate fields (crystallographers, x-ray diffractionists, biologists, biochemists).

In considering application of medical research we must return again to the field of human genetics, one which has accumulated a vast store of empirical observations relating to congenital malformations and diseases of childhood.* Much of observed data lack firm understanding among those who would risk using it

*The Committee on Human Genetics, World Health Organization, recommended recently that "Health" insurance cover cost of genetic counseling and related laboratory services; and stressed importance of establishing genetic counseling centers in those areas of the world where there is a high frequency of genetic blood disorders (sickle cell anemia and thalassemia). *Int. Med. News Service,* Vol. 12, No. 12 (December), 1969.

as a modality and language in the art of healing. The role of the professional genetic "counselor" therefore becomes problematical and the language of genetic counseling to date one of calculated risk in the advising and guidance of physicians and their patients.

Should there occur complete scientific understanding of results of research analysis in genetics or eugenics in the philosophy of medicine, the next step would be decision making as to extent of application of results to individuals or to society as a whole.

There are cumulative memories of the entire evolutionary process of mankind engraved in the genetic chemistry of humanity's common gene pool. As succeeding generations evolve, its members consciously or unconsciously to some extent relive experiences of preceding ones. Changes occurring in human and other organisms through the process of evolution make them either more or less adaptable to their environments. In this respect "mutations" may be "good" or "bad" depending upon whether or not they help the human organism survive its environment in present and succeeding generations.

Even when "mutation" is expressed in the tragic manifestation of mental deficiency or retardation deformity in a child at birth, one cannot be sure whether anticipatory adaptative processes in evolution are at work to create a greater number of automatons in the species with greater adaptability to man's technological "progress." It is conceivable that technology itself, especially in the visual media, could create its own automatons as an adaptive process among certain human beings.

If medicine is to play an increasing role in the field of genetics it must consider in its philosophy of research that the "random walk" of genes in the common pool has operated over generations not only in evolving problems but in their solution. In addition to those human beings who have evolved with inherited resistance to environmental problems such as heat, cold, hunger, infection, carcinogenecity, and other forms of stress, conceivably there are some whose ancestors lived on natural atomic piles and hence have inherited in their genetic chemistry resistance to radioactivity.

When man organizes medical research he must consider not only where mankind is at present and will be in the future but where he has been. A large modicum of reflective philosophical treatment seems indicated in dealing with what may be a harmonious balance between forces of free natural selection involving human migrations,* individual urges, and whims and those factors considered monitorable according to results of scientific analysis. Reflective treatment also is in order for other phases of medical research in disease prevention and control.

In other phases of medical research a number of paradoxes are created in solving problems at one end of life's spectrum, leaving greater and more pressing ones unsolved at the other. Perplexities of gerontology and geriatrics stem from the solution of problems in pediatrics and preventive medicine.**

Semantically the words *preventive medicine* are regarded in an ultimate sense as in the *prevention* of death, making man immortal. The words *geriatrics* and *gerontology* lose much of their meaning since these studies have become isolated from social context where the bulk of relevance lies. The research in these fields could yield even greater paradoxes than preventive medicine if inadequate consideration is made—geoeconomic, geodemographic, physiological, theological, and other implications.

From what has been discussed it seems important to medicine that those engaged in its scientific analyses have a broad conspectus of a million years in both the physical and cultural aspects of human history. In preoccupation with cases, patients, syndromes, and diseases, researchists cannot afford to lose sight of mankind as a whole. They must frequently ask, What is man? How did he get to be the way he is now, with his remarkable variety of attributes?

*Many geneticists and cultural anthropologists claim these too may be influenced by individual genetic "drives" separating those content to remain from those who wish to leave or escape town, city, or homeland.

**Of equal importance, in the saving of lives, was the development of occupational hygiene and safety programs at places of work; these programs saved untold millions of adult workers from disability and premature deaths through monitoring and control of occupational hazards.

In influencing man's evolution by discovery the scientist, the medical researchist, carries on his analyses not in a vacuum but within the confines of and subject to the practices of the polity. It is within the polity that arrangements and determinations are made concerning not only man's general mode of commonality but how the results of scientific analysis are to be put to use. When we speak of ethical codes in medical research involving both its methods and the application of its discoveries, we are really speaking of the requisites and regulations of society. Only insofar as medical ethics conform with these requisites can newly discovered powers in medicine be applied to society. For example, the fundamental canon of medical ethics, *Primum non nocere* (First of all do no harm), becomes ambiguous today in light of the new techniques in surgical transplantations. Because of possible divided loyalties of physicians toward either the donor or recipient, society requires answers to the questions, To whom should no harm be done? Who is dead and who is not?

Historically the healing art has opposed vociferously custody of its ethics by society, since it considered society poorly qualified to judge moral proprieties in medical practice or research. Medicine's premise has been that the polity is guided by emotionalism and those in research, by rational analysis. This dubious dichotomy proposes that emotionalism precludes rationalism and vice versa. Admittedly scientific analysis and discovery are important instruments in man's evolution, taking him from barbarism to "civilization" (or from one form of civilization to another). In the future, however, as in the past, medical or other research cannot hope to escape guidance and censure by the master arranger of man's affairs, the polity.

We must question not only relevance of Hippocrates' *Primum non nocere* but Bernardian limits on human experimentation. Claude Bernard proposed a medical and surgical "morality" based on the "duty" and "rights" of the medical profession to perform experiments on man whenever these experiments can save his life, cure him, or "gain him some potential 'benefit.' "

Bernard admonished those in medical research never to perform a harmful experiment on man even though results might be highly "advantageous to science," in other words, to the health of others. He adds that "performing experiments and operations exclusively from the point of view of the patient's advantage does not prevent their turning out profitably to science." Ambiguity here lies first in what duties or rights does the medical or any other profession have other than those bestowed by society, and secondly, are *potential* benefits synonymous with declared or undeclared "self-interests" of the patient? Also, are the self-interests of the patient totally defined in terms of his physiological integrity? The social order continues to affirm that medical or other types of scientific analysis cannot serve as an end in itself, even as the means for preserving life, unless its results enable individuals to live lives more than ones of biological longevity or physiological integrity. Whenever scientific analysis threatens the dignity and freedoms considered appropriate to man, the polity sooner or later makes proscriptions against this endeavor.

If we abandon Hippocratic and Bernardian principles, where can we turn for canons suitable to medicine's philosophy and its organization of medical research and its experiments?

The more philosophical medical researchists, in light of recent discoveries, have given thought to ethical criteria of research based on moral, legal, sociological, and theological terms. Historically, physicians have refused to make judgments as to the "worthiness" of this or that patient to receive the benefits of medical care in "moralistic" or theological frames of reference. The word *moral* has a varied impact on varied people according to their social or theological awareness. Semantic nuances make for difficulties in describing a philosophy of medical research in strictly moralistic or theological terms.

So far in this writing, medicine's philosophy has been considered mainly without theological points of reference. These cannot be ignored since the social order has for a great part of its history prescribed them in one form or another in the conduct of human affairs.

In the organization and methodology of medical research some investigators have proposed a basis in the canon of general ethics for all communal living. Originating in the social order and relating as it does to husbandry of material possessions; conventional requirements; and family, national, and international and other forms of social behavior, this canon would certainly give a broad and seemingly valid basis for ethical considerations in medical research. Its semantic impairment lies, however, in that it emanates from the *golden rule* and therefore is suitable in application to physician-patient relationships in medical research and practice. The rule as usually stated is a Christian positive restatement of the ancient Rabbi Hillel's negative command, "Do not unto others as you would not have them do unto you." In its Christian and positive form it is thought be be, by some scholars, a perversion leading to justification of self-righteousness and authoritarianism.

When we speak of the golden rule we have arrived at a juncture where we find man living both horizontally and vertically, with considerable tension at the intersection. It is from this tension that man's theological thinking often emerges. While what is called the golden rule is a principle of conduct that can and has existed outside of strictly theological points of reference, it has had its clearest definition and acceptance (in word or spirit) in the various formal religions of mankind. It was found early among the values of Hebrew and Christian tradition. It was present in the minds and writings of those who did atrocious medical experimentation in the prison camps of Hitlerite Germany. It is ubiquitous in spoken language but in action mutable according to chimerical needs of people, their cultures, and societies. It frequently dismays those who attempt to relate to or identify with it, since many, having lost inner capacity to affirm, are unable to accept this or other ethical principles as real or powerful attributes within themselves. This is often manifested by a "neutrality" of feelings toward issues not only among individuals but whole societies.

History attests to religiousness as an inalienable part of human nature, and perhaps in the sense that all men at some time in their lives deal with matters of "ultimate concern" they are all religious. Counter to these inclinations are forces of modernity. Some fear that modernity will cause man's religion to disappear altogether from the world. Others fear the opposite—religion becoming too successful and unrestrained. While admittedly man's discovery and invention become distractions in pursuit of religiousness he has in the main evolved adjustments and adaptations in language and action so he can take part in two worlds, or two aspects of the same world. So too the *Risorgimentos* of religion give evidence to their own evolution. Processes occurring in the realm of man's spirituality often produce ethical positions available and many times useful to the social order. So far religiousness in some form or other has weathered the storm of man's modernity. The contradictions man has placed in his heart and mind continue to motivate belief in the presence of a "superintending" force in the world and his sonship to that force.

Man willfully can and has, both in ancient and modern history, separated himself from dependency on theological and ethical norms but found the price, in resulting dehumanization, too great a threat to social homeostasis (the threat from within mankind). Expedients leading to dehumanization historically have been measured by concurrently evolving ethical positions produced by theological systems of thought. Present systems give encouragement to scientific and technical efforts on the part of man including efforts aimed at domination over nature. Expedients affecting social and moral orders of man will continue to be largely interdicted.

Within a hierarchy acting as custodian for theological and ethical values, the golden rule as an ethical canon for medical research may have validity in the preservation of human dignity. At individual case levels, however, its validity would depend on each practitioner's sense of authoritarianism and self-righteousness as a humanitarian. This could have overtones of euthanasia, regardless of society's proscriptions. It would be the medical scientific community's prime responsibility to exercise ethical control over individual situations. Control is not easily or properly exacted by rigid formulation of laws or injunctions, but is prompted by the heart speaking of *caritas* and benevolence— qualities medical investigators and practitioners should possess. In the organization of medical research today, the language

should be one of love and reverence for life, intimately bound
with ultimate aims of physicians in medicine's philosophy.

The Government of Medical Research

Under organization of research, mention was made of economic language spoken in its administration. Alluded to was the important role of research funding by government and private foundations of teaching and other medical institutions. In more recent years the pharmaceutical industry also has joined in this supportive sponsorship of medical research. This has increased numbers of researchists in medical teaching institutions if not the number of good teachers or practitioners.

The chronic financial insolvency of most medical schools precipitated their participation in sponsored medical research, which as will be seen became both a boon and a burden. In keeping with American character, Pegasus, steed of Aesculapius, is tied to one bandwagon or another where medical research may languish.* In bondage, medical research becomes victim of whims and foibles inherent to profit-motivated endeavors of drug manufacturers, personal disease interests of prominent personalities in government or elsewhere, and structured economic or other interests of research foundations. While much good has been accomplished, as in the case of vaccines developed for infectious diseases, the administration of research in the field of drug development has at times been productive of results that have rightly been termed "unspeakable."

Government policy on research in the medical sciences is torn by the "vested" interests in disease research.** These involve

*See de Chardin, Teilhard, *The Phenomenon of Man* (Organization of Research).

**Until 1949, the federal government took little interest in financing medical research (except for the Children's Bureau). This indifference was shaken, strangely enough, by the launching of a Russian Sputnick in 1957; at this time, President Eisenhower created the post of an assistant in his office on matters of science and technology. This post included some responsibilities for advising the President on biomedical sciences.

many persons who make a professional way of life by promoting one form of disease, giving it higher priority for research funds than another; i.e., cardiovascular disorders versus cancer or hereditary diseases and deficiencies versus arthritis and emphysema. Until recently largely ignored have been problems created by man (environmental health hazards and problems in social science).

An area of public controversy involves diversion of government research funds from "direct" research in "conquests" of specific diseases (cancer, heart disease, arthritis, neuromuscular disease) to "indirect" research; i.e., that of creating a "knowledge establishment" in biomedical research. Here, the term knowledge establishment refers to medical schools that on the whole are in dire financial straits and accept biomedical research as a means of general financial support of basic graduate and professional education functions. If this be a ruse it is one of necessity.

The analogy here would be of a baker willing to buy the most expensive ingredients for his icings but no flour for his cakes. Government has been willing under public pressure to purchase the most expensive types of medical research but has not given sufficient direct support until recently to institutions of higher professional learning.

While biomedical science has become inextricably woven to the fabric of medical education, public awareness of specific deficiencies in medical knowledge and service is out of proportion to its awareness of the crucial needs of medical education in money and manpower. Basic needs of education, biomedical research, and the public must all be served.

Adding to the confusion in the governing of research is a large professional class of politically wise entrepreneurs (the gunslingers of science) whose scientific skill becomes subordinated to aims not primarily in the interest of seeking scientific truth.* They introduce into research an element of super-salesmanship.

*The "scientific" muckrakers picture these individuals as maneuvering in a corrupt fashion for the scientific dollar. Weinberg, Alvin. "In Defense of Science." *Science* (Jan. 9), 1970.

This is directed at garnering research funds for schools and other institutions they represent. Their techniques are similar to those of professional militarists who revert to civilian life and obtain government armament contracts for industrial concerns. Some of these individuals have strained the credulity of the polity and its government by overplaying "politics of promise."

As in protocols and contracts, the language of research administration becomes predominantly economic rather than scientific. Government monies become "labeled" for types of scientific analyses considered *germane* to government's mission. Both legislative and executive branches of government decide which goals in research are more useful, productive, "worthy," and necessary. National priorities are set in research development and application. This burden to government has become great, so great that addition of a new cabinet seat called "Secretary of Science" has been advocated.

Grants received from government by individuals or institutions bring on responsibilities in fields of personnel administrations; also to be considered are civil rights, patent and copyright policies of the government, provisions of the Animal Welfare Act, conflict of interest clauses, budgets, and cost accounting and myriads of financial control procedures. In this manner able investigators become constrained in scientific endeavor, and qualifications other than scientific competence are asked of them.

Government judgments concerning medical and other research cannot be escaped. As indicated, direction of this research has become a matter of national policy. However, even with this framework, the best interests of society will not always be served since neither scientists nor government always know in advance to what use results of scientific discovery will be put. Only when statecraft fits requirements of medical and other research into patterns of social responsibility the best interests of the polity are most apt to be served.

In medical research conformity to governmental administration can be detrimental first to the language and later the behavior of those engaged in research. While the fruits of science are presumed to be morally neutral, scientists under the aegis of government frequently find themselves holding either formal or informal public image and authority. Their language as scientists can become lost in a mire of platitudes and contingencies. Issues are debated by scientists claiming the immunity of "objectivity" from social judgments; at times the same scientists will argue their qualifications to make *social judgments* in matters involving scientific discovery and its application to society.

It is of great interest semantically that the "crisis facing American science" was described as resulting from the enactment by Congress of the Revenue and Expenditure Control Act of 1968.* Here within the context of inflationary control we see benefits of medical research treated economically and more as a luxury than an activity essential to society.

It can be argued that conformity to a commissariat governmental effort in coordinating national goals and priorities in the administration of medical research would damage pure scientific initiative and stifle the "free-wheeling" inventive genius, which in the past has furnished successful responses to problems of research. Even the most ascetic of those in pure basic research may become infected with economic language. Few can remain islands of neutrality when confronted by vast amounts of literature circulated in academic circles concerning government research budgets.

Scientists working under government contracts are asked to "allocate" reductions, submit revised budgets, and make recommendations on how to defer expenditures of current budgetary allotments in keeping with recommendations of governmental bodies. Surely those with a sincere interest in scientific analysis suffer traumatic distraction from dedication and self-sacrifice. Under these conditions the exaction of laboratory work may cease to be looked on as a joy by the scientist or as a service to humanity. These administrative techniques requiring skills other than scientific frequently determine the economic status of those engaged in the research. The professional lives of those in medical

---

*Recent appropriations bills passed by Congress (1969-1970) are even more restrictive and curtail sharply expenses allowable for basic medical research.

research can be affected by economic language of contracts. Thus the contract system, which is an important invention by government in administering medical research, not only becomes a nationalizing influence of private sectors of medical research; it affects the language and action of scientists who must employ its administrative techniques.

Economic structuring is prominent elsewhere in research: to some degree in its administration by private, nonprofit, or charter foundations; to a greater degree in wholly commercial research institutions, particularly those in the pharmaceutical industry. We have in these latter instances potential corrupting influences on the morality and language of medicine.

The commercial development of medication designed to heal the sick flourishes in an economic climate tempered by government labeling regulations. A large "adversary" system of medical scientific analysis and data collection has developed to protect vested interests of manufacturers. Involved at times as adversaries are segments of the research industry including government; drug manufacturers; and municipal, state, and federal regulatory bodies. Manufacturers usually with intellectual honesty, albeit with some human observer "parallax" attempt to justify benefits of products in relation to potential or calculated risk of harm to the public.

In instances, through ill advisement, human parallax, or economic reasons, manufacturers may become true adversaries of the social order. To the extent that the healing art becomes a part of this adversary system, the art becomes corrupted in the governing of its research. This can be especially degrading to medical practitioners and educators either receiving financial support from or serving as policy-making members of drug corporation boards. Conflict of interest may develop when these practitioners are called upon to participate in the clinical evaluation of drugs.

To a lesser extent the financial support derived from drug industry advertising and loaned to physicians for their organizations or publications can become demoralizing.

It appears that the language of the adversary systems of medical information, whether it is in medical research, occupational medicine, or jurisprudence, becomes a corrupting influence inimical to the higher goals of the healing art. It is conceivable that the social order will in the foreseeable future declare this and other aspects of medicine out of bounds to the usual profit motivations of industry. This is suitable to a new philosophy in medicine and the great works expected of it in the future. Further, it seems patent in the protection of its integrity that practitioners support public efforts in instituting national independent drug testing, which gives anonymity to the drug manufacturer.

A recent semantic problem in medical research relates to joint efforts of industry and medicine in biomedical engineering. The problem involves interplay in awareness, and language becomes a barrier in research development. Medicine and engineering are jointly involved in development of computer diagnosis, medical instrumentation, and systems analysis in delivering health services to population groups. In such joint efforts there are mutual expectations sometimes based on disorganized concepts of one discipline relating to another. The engineers find that those in biological and medical sciences, especially educators, lack "drawing-board" skills and awareness and at times precision in record keeping and sophistication in mathematics, both *sine qua nons* in engineering. On the other hand biomedical scientists expect engineers to develop structures or instrumentations more closely resembling some scheme of nature; they find it difficult to accept mechanical models proposed by the engineers, which although mathematically good pumps or other devices, have deficiencies when applied to problems of human physiology.

Medical researchists live with continued hope and expectation that tomorrow will bring still better equipment but more in the image of nature's designs. In this manner the medical-industrial alliance in research has pitfalls in communication. Motivated by profit incentive, industry's engineers, efficiency, and new technologies can serve the cause of medical research; on the other hand there is obvious merit in the expectations of those in medical education and research. While man in his present state has acquired excellence in mathematical calculation—let's say of the critical angle in a pumping mechanism—he is still often unable to match the mathematical accuracy that evolution has produced in design of a human kidney or heart. It may be undesirable therefore to modify the awareness and language of those in medical research to any degree of total consonance with that of engineering and mathematics.

Reports of research activity in medicine's own journals give evidence that medical research already may have leaned too far in the direction of adopting the language of mathematicians and physicists. As an example, the word "parameter"* has the ring or impact of fundamental mathematical and physical science, not just of biological or medical science. Some medical writers prefer (as a matter of prestige) publication in journals of science, biological and physical, and eschew what they consider less scientific and less erudite medical journals. In attempting to impart an air of erudition to published papers (and to themselves) in the eyes of mathematician and physicist as well as physician friends, they will "borrow" the language of these friends. They may be unaware that a word, "parameter," is used in a most precise fashion by theoretical physicists and mathematicians. Parameters were used in their "broadest" context by Einstein in proving mathematically uniformity in the speed of light in all directions by application of Lorenzt Transformation formula to Cartesian geometric coordinates. In recent years we find in medical literature blood counts, blood pressure, serum cholesterols, weights, heights, and even age and sex described as "parameters." The questions here are not only whether the term within its present mathematical definition is debased by its use in medicine but what is happening in the behavior of those in medical research who employ the term to lend "scientific dignity" to their reports.

Hopeful indeed was the response within organized medicine to the need for unrestricted grants in the administration of research so that monies would be available for needs as determined by recipients rather than donors. That this response proved a successful technique is evidenced by governmental agencies' accept-

*An arbitrary constant characterizing, by each of its particular values, some particular member of a system of expressions, curves, surfaces, and functions.

ance of it to a degree through the process of mimesis. Whether the efforts of organized medicine to establish an unfettered system of grants to medical education and research will have the same success depends to a large measure on the reliance placed on receipts of donations from sources outside the healing art. Funds of this nature coming from industries, especially those in the pharmaceutical field, could present difficulties. On the whole, however, the greater the involvement of organized medicine in the professional planning and administration of its research and teaching the greater the expectation for fulfillment of results consistent with its future great tasks.

In reviewing the organization and governing of medical research we find that if the medical profession's responsibility is to be genuine in this field it must be exercised fully in establishing policy and standards for its own research and development. Further, it must not allow the language of other disciplines, including those involving husbandry, to cloud its scientific horizons and objectives. Above all it should exercise a morality in its research consonant with patterns of existing social responsibility by setting standards for conduct of research to protect the integrity of the profession, its members, and society. In exercising this morality, the objectives of its research would be to create a more livable world and, as Dr. Alvin Weinberg has stated, "to restore man to a state of balance with his environment; to resolve the remaining elementary and primitive suffering of man—hunger, disease, poverty, and war." These are neither simple nor new tasks for the healing art but must become articles of faith.

CHAPTER IV

Bennett, Miriam F. "The Clock and the Calendar of the Earthworm." *Zeitschrift für Vergleichende Physiologie,* 60:34, 1968.

Beveridge, W. I. B. *The Art of Scientific Investigation.* London: William Heineman Ltd., 1950.

Burrow, Trigant. *Science and Man's Behaviour.* New York: Philosophical Library, 1953.

de Chardin, Teilhard. *The Phenomenon of Man.* New York and Evanston: Harper & Row, 1961.

Fast, Howard. *The Jews—Story of a People.* New York: Dial Press, 1968.

Frank, Philipp. *Modern Science and its Philosophy.* Cambridge: Howard University Press, 1941.

Luria, Salvador E. *Medical Tribune Report.* "The New Science of Genetic Engineering." (November 17), 1969.

Mintz, M. F. and Panalba, D. A. "A Conflict of Commercial, Therapeutic Goals." *Science* (Aug. 29), 1969.

Mraca, Gene L. "Research Progress Forward on Artificial Hearts." *Modern Medicine* (November 17), 1969.

"The New Science of Genetic Engineering." *Report* (November 17), 1969.

Oppenheimer, J. Robert. *Science and Common Understanding.* New York: Simon and Schuster, 1953.

Stover, Carl F. The Government of Science—A Report to the Center For Study of Democratic Institutions. Santa Barbara, California: The Fund for the Republic, 1962.

Weinberg, Alvin. "In Defense of Science." *Science* (January 9), 1960.

Young, J. Z. *Doubt and Certainty in Science.* London: Oxford University Press, 1951.

CHAPTER V

Present Language of Dispute

in the Delivery of Medical Care

In all language the need for specificity of meaning arises as a semantic requirement of communication. Philosophers describe, in the abstract, birth, life, and death as "accidental phenomenal" attributes of the flowing "substrate" of mankind and all living things. The man or patient we speak of, however, is the "now" and "here" man of flesh and bone, desiring immortality and afraid to die. His reason tells him he must, but the *soma* of his bowels and muscles refuse "reason." He is the man whose body in youth seemed at one with the spirit but in old age appears at war. No amount of anticipatory preventive or curative medicine now or in the future will offer permanent relief for this feeling deep down inside of man.* While we can optimistically predict, to a degree, increasingly greater longevity for him with greater physical comfort, we cannot give him the breadth and depth at the end of his life's spectrum as at the beginning. Perhaps we need as much cultural skill in teaching men how to die as in conserving their life spans.**

*Notwithstanding the parroting of "an ounce of prevention, etc." and the Greek adage, "Help people die young as late as possible."

**Freud once remarked that "Our attitude toward death includes a denial of its happening, to ourselves or loved ones; when it does so with the latter, it is imputed to accident or disease; never to inevitability."

Born with impairment inherent in his sense of mortality, the threat, real or imagined, of affliction by disease can become an alienating, ego-crushing experience to man. Whether he be a farm laborer or board chairman, disease is an attack on his self-concept. As a patient he seeks the physician as one of the last bastions of nonaggressiveness, placing the entire responsibility for the discovery of illness in his hands. While at times he may, consciously or unconsciously, semantically block communication of those thoughts and feelings that may facilitate the diagnosis of his ills, he expects the physician to search for, find, and remove the threat to his ego.

The alienation effect of severe illness can make all men "marginal" and irrelevant to the mainstream of human existence, in the same sense as the monk, the displaced person, the prisoner, and all those persons who live in the presence of misery and death. Reinhold Niebuhr once remarked,

> "What about man, this strange and pathetic individual, who is so insignificant in the coherences and incoherences of nature and of history and so significant to himself and to the people who love him? . . . What are you going to do with the pathos of individual existence? And what are you going to answer when he asks the question 'What is the meaning of my individual and my collective destiny anyway'?"

This same man is depicted today a "consumer" of medical services. He has certain expectations as a consumer in those matters pertaining to services he receives. He may expect that he, not the office or hospital personnel, embodies the *raison d'être* of the service establishment. Though sympathetic to the cause of medical science, as a consumer usually he has no expectations of being a text or case for research or teaching purposes. He expects advantages of modern diagnosis and therapy to alleviate or cure his illness, but not substituted disease syndromes or complexes as a result of therapy.

The human being as a patient, with an ego already impaired by illness, by nature becomes defensive regarding all verbal symbolic language of action and arrangement in medical care. We must consider each human being as an individual whose particular response to pain expresses his nervous system's unique codification of stimuli. The same applies to body responses to disease processes where a "little" disease causes an unexpected response in morbidity while in another individual the same or greater amounts of disease may be asymptomatic. Therefore some individuals differ in body language from others, which makes individualization in treatment of paramount importance.

While much consideration is being given to quantitative problems in delivery of medical care, comparatively little is paid to qualitative aspects of medical care to *individuals*. Humanity's needs in relief of pain and misery historically have been met in a discriminatory fashion. Too often in medicine's philosophy, rights by virtue of race, class, creed, or financial circumstances become determinants in the quality of medical care delivered. In this area of human need, as in the Spanish tradition, all men are nobles, equal to the king though their wordly goods be less than the king's. The best medical care available in a particular society would seem the right of every individual member. This would include even those "single-purpose" individuals who may live mainly on the labors of others and wastrels whose own self-neglect may have contributed to their disease state.

Those who are cured, survive, or adapt to the severe stress of mental or physical illness, no matter how badly they act in the sickroom or ward, are heroic and deserve to be so regarded by other members of society. They perhaps deserve freedom from economic fears, phobias, and anxieties as tributes to their heroism. Their "cause" as individuals who have suffered the alienation of illness, disability, or despair on the battlefield of life is as noble as if suffered in military conflict.

Much of the language of dispute on the subject of medical care among practitioners, their patients, and the social order centers on economics and the rights and privileges of practitioners versus the rights and privileges of human beings generally. While refusing to be casuistic in other phases of their art, many practitioners today consider good medical care a privilege—a privilege to be earned, in the protestant or puritan ethical sense, through hard work and prudence in the planning and saving of financial resources.

Again in the philosophy of medicine we face the concept of rewards to man, considered due him only through his industry applying not only to his wants but primitive needs. If man wishes to "profit" from medical care, the physician, the insurance industry, the drug industry, the hospital, all must profit from the patient's diligence, hard work, and prudence. This makes him a "consumer," and cost-of-living indices reflect both his wants in goods and needs in medical care. Thus misery is compounded by the pious accountancy under the ethic of work and reward. The degree of humaneness inherent in this system of delivery of medical care is questionable in a philosophy of medicine designed to meet great future tasks.

Service plans and systems of indemnification for medical and hospital expense (erroneously termed "health insurance") ring with language of arms-length bargaining and the virtues and ethos of the profit system. In the guise of "benefit" plans they are built upon pooling of risk and contain self-protective limitations and exclusions, which can adversely affect coverage in the very cases of illness needing coverage most. As in other aspects of insurance the true nature of coverage purchased may be obscured by language based on juxtaposition of words, technicalities of underwriting, and limited attention given to contract provisions by the purchaser.* The medieval principle *caveat emptor*, found in darker areas of business, still has application to the selling and buying of medical and hospital insurance.

In a mobile society where frequent change of employment is common, persons having suffered an illness or injury at one place of employment may find effects of the same illness specifically excluded from future coverage, in a new individual policy or group insurance plan. These are individuals frequently most in

---

*The lack of insurance coverage for many clinical tests related to thorough diagnostic procedures may be unknown to both physician and his patient until later ruled upon by the insurance carrier.

need of coverage who may suffer catastrophic medical and hospital expense. In insurance of medical care, therefore, whether it be for professional services of a physician, hospitalization, or purchase of medication, the principle of *caveat emptor* in insurance becomes inappropriate and may leave the insured defenseless against the onslaught of a particular illness, perhaps for a lifetime.

Increased costs in delivery of medical care has resulted from more recent advancements in medicine and surgery, such as kidney transplants. These costs, well out of reach for the average patient, also have caused insurance companies to reconsider methods of pooling risks. The need for restructuring and spreading of risks and premium costs involved in these new therapeutic techniques could well place present systems of voluntary prepaid medical insurance in a state of continuing obsolescence. Whether the insurance industry, faced with even greater advancements in medicine and surgery, can remain competitive on a profit-incentive, free-enterprise basis has been questioned.

In periods of retrospection following medical breakthroughs, the social order clamors for the common good in its wants and needs regardless of economic or other obstructions *(summum bonum)*. This clamor becomes intensified by legitimate demands for public information, which at times, corrupted with careless and sensational publicity, creates false hopes among a great number of the sick. Medicine and journalism alike share casuistic responsibility in scientific matters when matters of hope and caution *(caveat venditor)* are without warrant couched in language purporting expectations to be realities.

Most of the dispute in the healing art today has its origin in modes of insurance protection for medical care and hospitalization. That its own language of dispute has in a semantic sense been at times catastrophic to it and its public image has become evident to many medical practitioners as well as to other members of the social order. Many practitioners over the years had reservations and doubts that the cure for this malady lay in political action by organized medicine.

Medicine in the United States was threatened with governmental intervention (Wagner, Murray, Dingell Bill)* to cure social and economic ills at a time when it was waging an unsuccessful crusade against voluntary prepayment medical insurance plans. In this setting extraordinary events occurred, steeped in politics and economics, with organized medicine and government adversaries. Having been cited by government (under the antitrust law) for prejudicial actions against practitioners affiliated with voluntary health insurance plans, organized medicine reluctantly accepted this form of insurance after being labeled by government as a "business" or "trade."

While some in the profession credit organized medicine with the espousement of voluntary prepaid insurance, this form of insurance was gradually accepted by the profession as the lesser of two evils. The greater evil was the threat to its security and homeostasis posed by legislation that would nationalize and monopolize insurance for medical care and hospitalization. Developments since place the profession in the unenviable position of fighting a continual rear-guard political action against society's pressuring for suitable responses to its medical care needs.

Since the healing art entered into dispute with social forces, much has changed in its language. Semantic problems, based on medicine's self-concept versus public image, unfolded with the profession feeling unloved. The social order, in labeling medicine a trade, was deemed unappreciative of all medicine had done for mankind. Meanwhile its communications and features of organization became such as to imply that the profession had been affected semantically by what it considered a degrading label.

There began, in the art of healing, a transition from guild professionalism to a form of syndicalism. The profession in dialogue with the public began to speak of legislative platforms, goals, and its need for medical statesmanship. In the realm of economics those in organized medicine spoke of parities between the products of industry and the "product" of medical care—

*The late John D. Dingell, Sr. (father of the present congressman from Michigan) in 1943 incorporated into his bill proposals once labeled socialistic—some of these proposals since have become law (federal support for medical research, hospital construction, aid to disabled, rural health plans).

this in terms of its purchase under market-dominated conditions. This implied that medical care, as part of a system of free enterprise, must above all be practiced on the basis of sound economic principles.*

The analogy drawn between provision of health services and conventional marketplace economy presents serious semantic difficulties since it exposes a multitude of differences among those that are free to "shop" for articles in the marketplace and those seeking medical care in a "nonbuyer's" market. The situations involved defy equation. One buyer is free to seek an article that will provide him most satisfaction at a price the buyer is willing to pay, as clothes, services, even food. The "buyer" or seeker of health services, emotionally charged by threat to his own or the security of loved ones, by contrast must and often with a feeling of urgency seeks medical care, as a matter of expediency, in a narrow or closed market.

Market theory provides that supply reacts reasonably promptly in response to variations in demand. This plainly is not the case, either with regard to the supply of physicians or their services.

There is also the question raised in the analogy as to whether in the marketing of goods we are referring to human "need" goods as much as to human "wanted" goods. The supply of medical care more often is related to human needs than wants. This is in contrast to the economic demand in marketing of goods based on ability to pay.

Later the profession came close to pronouncing semantic absolution and death on itself as an art in testing its latent tendencies toward syndicalism. Threats to withhold services from the public were made and carried out in a province of Canada and other countries of the world. It is to the credit of those creative minorities in organized medicine in the United States, responding to public anxiety and apprehension, that the language of syndicalism was not carried to its logical extension in boycotts and

*One large organization of specialists (pathologists) had as one of its important objectives promotion of business-management training courses among its members as a logical step in dealing with present-day methods of computer accounting.

strikes. These minorities saw and overcame a threat within the ranks of medicine, which could have destroyed the profession semantically as a healing art.

Enlightened practitioners saw in the logical context of syndicalism the emergence of language with serious unfavorable impact on the profession's public image. It became obvious to organized medicine that syndicalistic language commonly employed lacked benignity and on the whole was unpalatable. Physicians generally, though restating their privileges as professional men, and not as tradesmen or a proletariat, saw no inherent rights in these privileges granted by society to boycott needs of humanity or laws of governments.

In its transition to greater awareness of social values, we find in medicine many more dedicated practitioners (especially recent graduates) willing to speak out against the status quo. Some of these have known extreme poverty and misery among patients. In the tradition of Schweitzer and other humanitarian philosopher-physicians in the history of medicine, some are less affected by the mores of the marketplace. There are those who would forego financial and social comfort—even their medical knowledge, practices, and licenses—rather than be associated with syndicalism in the art of healing. Many consider the privilege exercised in the practice of medicine philosophically to be a cardinal act of mercy. Their dissatisfaction with stereotyped reactionary responses within organized medicine to challenges in medical care portends an important influence for change in the philosophy among many succeeding generations of practitioners.

It was fortunate for medicine that revolt occurred within its ranks. The dominant majority was required to reexamine its philosophy and language and its present-day relevance to greater and more valuable goals.

Relevance of certain Hippocratic principles to modern medicine came under question. Creative minorities in medicine had found Hippocrates' oath to carry out a regimen for the sick and "to keep them from harm and wrong" being fulfilled in words but not in spirit. The Hippocratic fulfillment had become clouded by language that exhorts physicians *not* to dispose of their services under certain terms or conditions. This includes conditions tending to interfere with or impair free and complete exercise of their medical judgment and skill and conditions generally that tend to cause a deterioration of quality of medical care. These norms are fraught with value judgments and semantic difficulties and become at times exercises in hypnopedagogics, Hegelian dialectics, producing obscurities in meaning and intent.

Regardless of the number of those in favor or against "free" hospitalization and medical care, organized medicine has consistenly identified "free" care with deterioration of quality. The concept of some direct payment by the patient of a fee for service was and is still held by many physicians to be an important factor in the acceptance, appreciation, and efficacy of the therapeutic relationship. Some even propose the "essence" of the physician-patient relationship is one of "commercial" interest. Here, a "unilateral" agreement on the part of the physician seeks as its premise the desire of the patient to "reward" the physician. Syllogistically the proposal introduces the premise that in our society people relate to all services received *via* economics. The conclusion reached is that "free" medical care, for this society, would be detrimental to the patient-physician relationship; and *ergo* the relationship derives a good measure of its integrity from its present concept as a basically monetary arrangement.

This "quintessent cynicism" dictates seemingly logical propositions that "something for nothing" yields nothing to the recipient; further, those being healed either appreciate or benefit less in the absence of monetary expenditures on their part in the physician-patient relationship. Even if society were permeated with a philosophy of cynicism, there are many in medicine who would still believe there are a large number of human beings who appreciate tangible benefits, even when received without monetary expense.

At one time the medical profession looked with cynicism on colleagues who agreed to dispose of their services to institutions on a salary basis. These arrangements were held to be terms or conditions tending to interfere with or impair free and complete exercise of medical judgment. A corollary was that physicians in the "competitive" practice of medicine on the whole exercised better judgment and skill than salaried colleagues. This became untenable since a large number of advancements in professional skill and judgment were brought about by salaried colleagues performing research, teaching, and clinical duties in governmental and private institutions. Without salaried "noncompetitive" physicians it is hard to conceive how community and environmental health services as we know them today could exist.

Objections to salaried physicians, raised by organized medicine in the late nineteenth and early twentieth centuries in the interest of quality control of medical care, largely have disappeared. There was, at one time, concern especially for those captive colleagues practicing medicine within industrial corporations,* required to do the bid of management.

As medical care became more complex, the need for basing professional rewards on time rather than on units of service to individual patients became apparent. As already indicated medical tasks involving research, teaching, or community health, employing salaried physicians (time versus individual units of service) had proven successful. Further, it has been found even where clinical service to patients is a major task that rewards to physicians by salary have great advantages over fees, for both physicians and patients.

Closely allied to "free enterprise" in the economic philosophy of organized medicine has been the "freedom of choice" concept. This is considered fundamental to human freedom in a democratic society much in the same fashion as the right to vote. It does not always mean self-determination on the part of the patient in seeking a quantity or quality of service.

"Choice" is seldom made with full freedom, nor can it always be a knowledgeable or enlightened one. Certainly economics directly influence freedom of choice. The ghetto dwellers frequently call city hospital ambulances for any type of medical service. More affluent patients are taught by the medical pro-

*Though partially emancipated by its later alignment with the American public health movement, occupational medicine as practiced early in American corporations was born in slavery, among narrow dark corridors of insurance and workmen's compensation medicine.

fession to report to hospital emergency rooms for care of injuries
and illnesses, many times not of an emergency nature. The concept of freedom of choice has therefore become paradoxical in
private practice. The *any* physician (licensed doctor of medicine)
becomes substituted for the freedom of choice principle, once
zealously guarded by organized medicine in espousement of free
enterprise in private practice.

To the public "enlightened referral to a dependable physician"* has become more important than freedom of choice. This
spares many patients the unfair burden of being knowledgeable
in choice of a physician.

In mobile societies many persons have limited knowledge of
local health institutions or facilities and the community generally,
so the facilitation, with maximum convenience, becomes paramount to the patient in the delivery of services, whether these
be preventive or curative in nature. This places the physician
and his organizations in important roles in the dialogue with the
social order and nurtures his dedication to more tangential,
professional communications. This nurturement would require
freedom from concern on the part of individual practitioners for
their own priorities and material self-interests. In this connection
semantic blocks to communication in referrals remain most severe between institutional and noninstitutional physicians and
require resolution.

Once patient-physician relationships are established through
"choice" made by or for the patient, we must consider the "in-

*In a recent survey (1969) of medical students, physicians, and
patients it was found that the quality of dependability was most frequently mentioned as the element sought in the patient-physician relationship. (Loftus, Gregory T., Michigan State University, College of Human
Medicine.) In this survey, physicians stressed value judgments related to
follow-through on diagnosis and treatment; those on faculties stressed
ethical issues on terminal illness and on problems of over-commitments
of private practitioners' time. Students showed concern for both scientific
understanding and "psychologic" support to cases. "Para-medical" personnel when asked gave value judgments stressing realistic concepts in patient
care. Patients emphasized importance of the physician's availability to give
them time sufficient to make them "feel like persons." A similar survey
at the University of Utah disclosed greater emphasis on value judgments
in line with scientific acumen, expeditious diagnostic and therapeutic
regimens, and the qualities of intellectual honesty and that of leadership.

tegrity" of relationships. This integrity must be viewed within modern context of an increasingly impersonal dialogue between physician and patient. Overspecialization has placed more emphasis on the science than the art of medicine; there has been a decline in the importance of the patient-physician relationship in the minds of many patients.

The integrity of patient-physician relationships depends on factors common to all human confrontations.* Patients ask whether physicians recognize and respect them as individuals; physicians ask whether patients recognize and respect them in the same manner. The content of mutual expectations far exceeds the apparent simplicity of patient-"sees"-physician. Few if any confrontations induce full acceptance of one person for another. Alien forces act counter to his acceptance: the patient's fear and trepidation of the unknown; authoritarian or nonauthoritarian symbolism in the confrontation setting; and all the kinds of beliefs applicable to the healing art and related expectations.

In a sense beliefs are derived from habit and used to overcome doubt. Their essence lies in establishment of habituality, and they become distinguishable by the different modes of action to which they give rise. They may range from mores or folkways of national origin, which encompass taboos and various degrees of cynicism, to present-day attitudes toward any authoritarian symbol, whether on the broad basis of civil authority or the more narrow or personal basis of parental relationships.

Many beliefs affecting patients' expectations of the healing art are primitive in nature, the more primitive akin to the ancient Balkan beliefs in sacrificial stone rituals as cures for sterility. The less primitive are: You will catch your death of a cold in the wet snow; I believe I am going into labor and a taxi driver will take me to a hospital; My friends say Jewish or Japanese doctors are very conscientious and more highly skilled. These are shared by many people and are based on common experiences in various physical and social environments.

---

*The author is of the firm opinion that, unless in great pain or discomfort, seldom do most human beings wish to see a physician or be told what is wrong with them.

Some beliefs are primitive in character but independent of others' experiences, arising from deep personal conviction. (The last time I felt this way my blood sugar was high, and I went into a coma.)

Other beliefs derived from authority in society may be tentatively accepted by individuals, depending on their trust or distrust of a particular social order. (That public clinic down the street will be a good place for the children; The company medical department gives good emergency care.) Peripheral beliefs shared with authorities in the social order usually cause the individual to identify or relate to the order and its beliefs.

Many beliefs today lack any primary drive for the individual and are dynamic, easily changeable, and resolve into matters of "taste" for people or things. (I don't believe in doctors who have *too* good a bedside manner.)

All the mentioned beliefs operative within the framework of a physician-patient relationship can bring various degrees of acceptance and nonacceptance of one for the other and complicate mutual expectations in the relationship. Even a family practitioner, native born in a well-circumscribed rural community, may fail to meet the total profile of beliefs that a patient may carry in mind as a guide-map to his territory of interpersonal relationships.

The healer to various degrees is an authoritarian symbol: he may represent to the patient the authority figure or a father who was too strict; a boss who is a martinet; or some authority figure met in the military or in the police department. To the more educated, not so much the countenance of the healer but his known or visible certifications and licenses become bases for judgment. A segment of the less educated is prone to accept the healer's designation as a "doctor" regardless of whether this be a doctorate in allopathy, osteopathy, or the chiropractic profession. These and other revolving torques or concentric circles of awareness among patients can either reinforce or nullify their favorable mood and manner. Labels in forms of certificates, diplomas, and licenses may or may not be fundamental to a patient's mood or manner or beliefs.

We must speak also of the language of arrangement in institutional settings, inducing semantic forces within the patient that affect either favorably or unfavorably already established bias or beliefs. The individual healer at work may have little to do with patients' acceptance; unless by mood or manner he poses an obvious threat, he blends into institutional backgrounds. Acceptance therefore by the patient becomes based on an "institutional authoritarianism" symbol. The *locus* of the physician may qualify him.

Thus we see how value judgments of human beings become colored by myriad circles of awareness and experience that have little to do with the professional competence of the individual healer. What the profession considers a patient-physician relationship involves a number of factors beyond the purview of the healing art, which can diminish or impair its integrity.

Monetary values placed within the relationship serve to accentuate negative factors operating against a full integrity among patients, especially among those who in their beliefs also may distrust the social order and may be suspicious of economic arrangements promulgated therein. Illness, major or minor, can be to some degree catastrophic among most persons. In purchase of surcease, fears of "fee" may stifle tokens of goodwill toward the healer. The language of many patients in their relationship to the physician thus can become "clothed" by fear of fees or by projection into the future a pessimism born of uncertainty as to consequences of what remains basically an unknown relationship. Rarely can the relationship be fully friendly in the sense of being devoid of factors mitigating against self-priorities or -interests (economic or otherwise) of those concerned.

If we examine further some of the language of dispute in medicine both within its ranks and with social forces (termed by some in medicine as "governmental interventionists"), we see curious divisive meanings expressed as to the relationship of government, including those in the American Public Health Move-

*Until recently, this movement had become encumbered with *semantic* corruption by use of labels or titles for its membership; i.e. the authoritative connotation of "Health Officer" or "Surgeon Generals" who frequently are neither officers, surgeons, nor generals.

ment* and in social action, to the will of the people. In question is the trustworthiness of government in custody of people's mandate; also whether commitment to "welfare" is or is not a great curse in social policy. The rhetoric surrounding the devisiveness is steeped at one extreme with total distrust in the workability of any social policy or socialism and at the other "extreme" the belief, shared by a growing number within the profession, that in a democracy, government's role is legitimate in helping its citizens.

Those distrusting social policy consider commitment to it and welfare to be a ruse of professional political opportunities. Some conservative stereotypes in medicine continue to look upon their practices strictly as means of earning "bread." These would foster a spirit of what they consider "benign" syndicalism within the profession to keep it "free" from social action. They ask that government investigate "social security" and all subsequent social legislation with the view of bringing back "into the fold of private enterprise insurance" the majority of those elderly citizens now covered by government welfare programs.

Those believing government to have legitimate interests in the welfare of its citizenry claim that, as in the past, the healing art possesses a "nostalgic myopia," which explains its failure to meet changing demands of society. This myopia threatens its past image and future role in humanitarian endeavor. Further, they believe self-priorities and professional financial interests of physicians can only hasten the day of greater governmental regimentation of the profession.

From this intraprofessional dialogue a synthesis of seemingly antithetical points of view has evolved, together with a reawakening of language of humanitarianism in the profession. We see laissez-faire economic principles—long held a panacea for problems in delivery of medical care—crumbling rapidly.

Still contained in the language of organized medicine are outdated economic principles borrowed from a mistaken conception ot Darwinism used to bolster belief in systems of free enterprise. Here, biological principles are perverted into socioeconomics and ethics. Since Darwin did not speak of individual but of specie fitness, in its true meaning Darwinism, applied to the social problems of man, becomes socialistic even though the principles of biological and social evolution are strikingly different.

Creative minorities who represent a threat from within to organized medicine argue that economic relics of eighteenth and nineteenth century philosophy were responsible for naive "idealism" concerning free enterprise. Rejected is the phrase "political intervention" used by organized medicine in the context of government as some alien force imposed from without the polity. Substituted is the belief that constitutional democratic governments exercise authority given it by the people. In this, organized medicine is reminded that physicians cannot, short of anarchy, divorce in a dichotomous fashion professionalism from membership in a society having collective will.

The concept, long held, that good medical care must be "earned" by the recipients is under attack. The profession is reminded here that many in society and government consider medical care a guaranteed right, not a privilege, of every citizen.

Stereotyped conservatist practitioners continue to ask for better performance from medicine's "front office" as means of protecting the status quo of the profession. Those who propound reactionism ask leadership for greater efforts in effecting a more "coercive monopolistic" system within the profession to combat coercive monopolies by governmental systems. This isolationism, asking physicians to abdicate responsibilities to society, since it lacked benignity, was short-lived.

To date organized medicine's leadership has chosen realistically a synthesis of ideas embodying a compromise with the will of the polity. Under the "unifying force" of its organization, medicine offers leadership to all those *inside* and *outside* the profession concerned with the delivery of "quality care for all." Those on the outside would include "huge, monolithic labor, government, and other 'influence' groups." Those on the inside consist of organized, more dedicated "cohesive" patterns of physicians representing medicine's "character," interests, and abilities in contributing to human welfare. While language of "opposing forces" could impair intent, the synthesis seemingly fashions productive effort in medicine's leadership in response to the challenge of what has been termed a "nonsystem" of medical care. This effort would continue to associate the healing art with others outside of medicine whose prime interest also lies in the delivery of quality medical care for all. A great degree of the realism in the synthesis is inherent if not expressed in organized medicine's admission that it "cannot do it all alone."

Whether the present state of affairs will allow medicine to be any more receptive to further government subsidy of medical care will depend upon its continuing intramural dialogue. This dialogue involves internal forces of stereotyped conservatism and growing numbers of young medical students and practitioners in its ranks who identify themselves with liberal ideology.

Organized medicine has in the past obtained solace through the political victories of conservatism in government but learned that social forces continue at work regardless of declarations made in the public political climate. How well the profession assesses and deals with these forces will depend upon whether it considers them mainly a threat to its homeostasis or a new challenge to its leadership for new and more successful responses. What organized medicine terms the "huge monolith of labor" has been convinced for some time (prior to 1940) that nothing short of a "universal" federal health insurance plan will deliver quality medical care to all. A strong segment of labor is of the opinion that present and future problems in delivery of medical care are beyond the "capabilities" of the "private insurance industry." Further, they believe the present "health-care" system in the United States is disorganized, disjointed: "an antiquated and obsolete nonsystem." Labor describes its plan for medical care as being "universal" rather than "compulsory," avoiding connotation of "socialized medicine." Reassurances are given to organized medicine that physicians "will not work for the government." Some segments of labor consider those who oppose the use of instruments of government in solving basic human problems such as medical care to be lacking in intelligence, "primitive and irresponsible."

With a lexicon learned at the bargaining table, where synthesis from thesis and antithesis becomes a way of life, labor in social action can employ language that at the same time is inflammatory and emolient. This language on one hand invites through inflammatory responses medicine's ruling majority into the political arena where debate on issues of social action culminates; on the other it invites through emolience dissatisfied factions of creative minorities within medicine to continue efforts toward its "internal reformation."

Inevitably an "inflamed" commercial insurance industry will enter the dialogue and do so with the disadvantage of not knowing whether to retain or discard remnants of its humanitarian self-concept. Already charged with "profiteering" and incapability of meeting the health care "crisis," it must reorganize its self-concept as an industry and perhaps by clearly stating it is not a social or a welfare agency. With this new self-concept it may not survive its encounter in the political arena where debate on social action culminates. The question in debate in all probability will not be whether private insurance or private enterprise generally can provide economic protection for medical care more efficiently than government, but whether or not private insurance is in the "business" for profit in an endeavor that may soon be considered "out of bounds" for profit making. The disclaiming a profit motive in the pooling of risk, through "scientific calculation," to meet the promise of protection in policies, would seem to emphasize inadequacies of insurance or the free enterprise system generally in bringing quality medical care to all citizens, both "good" and "bad" risks. We may witness the disappearance of "actuarial calculism" from the languages of debate, a language organized medicine leaned heavily upon in defense of free enterprise in the delivery of medical care.

In ensuing controversy, regardless of repeated assurances from "adversaries" as to the excellence of American medicine, practitioners of the healing art still may be drawn into a "paranoid dream" where they may interpret the public's or labor's dissatisfaction based on economics as an attack on their medical competence. As among nations, the paranoid dream among individuals and groups of a society often produces misinformation reports, fallacious in judgment and inference, the logical extension of which is revenge among groups, which is the worst form of stress whether it be among members of a society or between nations. Within societies, crusades for "rights" frequently become indistinguishable from "revenge." The stress of attack on its self-concept, whether this concept is organized or disorganized, would produce a communicative deadlock between medicine and those outside of the profession, considered its adversaries. This would occur in the political debate among practitioners, labor, the polity, and its government. We can represent this communicative deadlock schematically. (See diagram on following page.)

The broken lines of stress shown throughout the diagram portray attempts by each side to change the other's organized self-concept of itself. In this process the communicative deadlock may create not only a vacuum of information but a growing nidus of misinformation to which the public becomes heir.

If organized medicine is to assume a posture of leadership in change, it may be required to abandon its historical conservatism in the ensuing social and ideological struggle. This may be difficult since justification of its conservatism has been based mainly on what was considered its inherent responsibilities (through Hippocratic relevance) to protect its tradition and the quality of medical care. Any effort or disposition toward preserving what is established will be labeled by opposing forces as an attempt at reversal in direction or manner of social progress, more specifically as reactionism.

Disposition of its opponents toward abrupt rather than gradual change in the character of medical care delivery will be termed "radical" and socialistic by organized medicine. As often happens, the dynamic nature of true democracy, which in logical extension becomes the world's most "radical" form of government, may go largely "unlabeled" or overlooked by both parties to the debate.

It appears that in the political arena the advantage lies on the side of the social forces, particularly labor, since their organized self-concepts in politics and social action, more nearly than organized medicine's, approach congruence with realities.

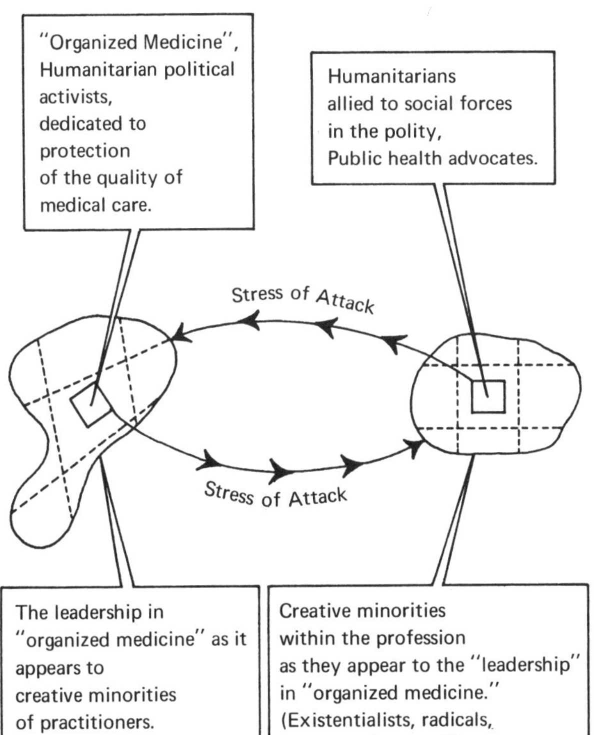

-------- Lines of stress and attrition when one side attempts to reorganize the self-concept of the other to conform to its own image of the other.

This may tempt medicine's organizational leadership to serve as an even greater single unifying political voice for practitioners, a role it has pursued in the past with ambivalence. To restructure its organized self-concept, giving clear and definite recognition to its new identity as an association of political power groups, might hasten culmination of the ideological struggle going on within its ranks. There would be problems of stress within its organization, which could impair unity in political action: As a result of this communicative deadlock within its own ranks, it is likely that the various city, county, and state components of organized medicine as well as the organizations already formed outside its ranks will become isolated from the main body and leadership.

In the meantime, in its quest for political advantage, organized medicine must continue to seek support from conservatives in government and its stereotyped counterparts in industry. Industry's responses no doubt will be in harmony with its own objectives and those of free enterprise, no matter how obnoxious those objectives are to labor and other forces of social action. These responses already propose application of industry's productive and manipulative scientific methods to the delivery of medical care. For example, one solution (termed by industry a "philosophy") to rapidly rising cost of continuing medical care proposes application of hotel-chain management skills to continuing care centers constructed adjacent to general hospitals.

Those in industry working with miracles of machine production, organization analysis, and computer technology possess philosophies relevant mainly to business, not community or social, environments. Having sold the public on its need for a wide variety of products, business and industry logically associate maximum service to the public with maximum long-term profit growth. In the environment of business beliefs, philosophies, and language are born that refuse to admit the stubborn facts of social policy and commitment. When challenged to sell itself to a large segment of society, which questions all present political and social tenets, industry is hard pressed to prove adequate social commitment. On one hand, industrialists realize that transition to new policies and philosophies are taking place; on the other they question with honesty and propriety industry's role as a social service agency.

As in other matters involving profit in collective enterprise we may find labor knowledgeable and equal to the task of discrediting efforts of an industry generally non-committed to solving social problems through profit growth. From long experience in bargaining for wages and working conditions, labor became as sophisticated as management concerning intracacies of "profit centers" and intracorporate competition among these centers. By the

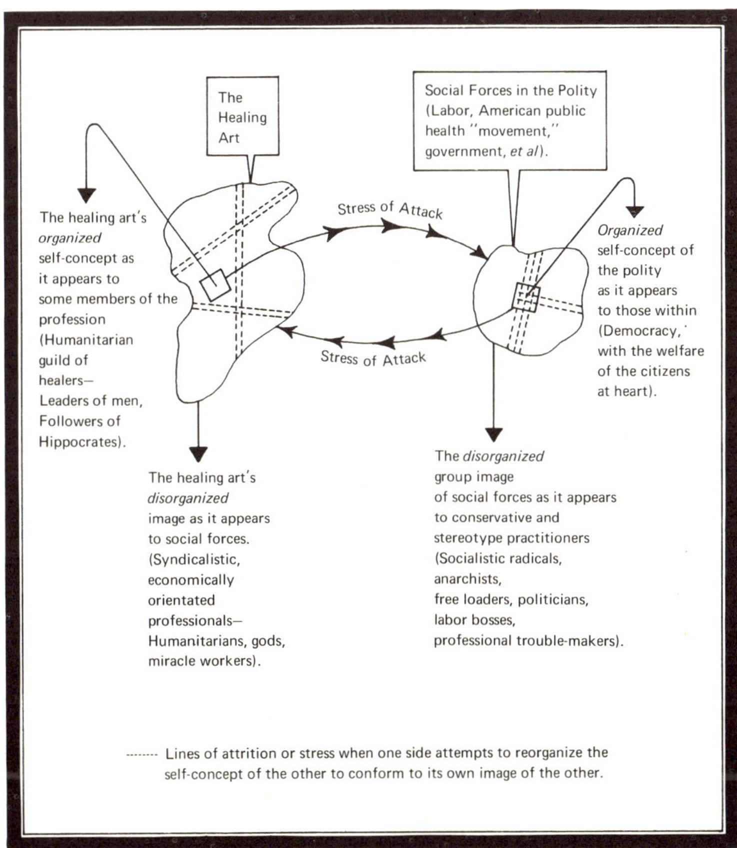

very inclusion of profit-center language into social debate, labor and other social forces gain an advantage in the discourse between themselves and the philosophy of those who speak the language of "pragmatic industrialism."

In the delivery of medical care we can further illustrate socio-economic forces and language at work in the following manner:

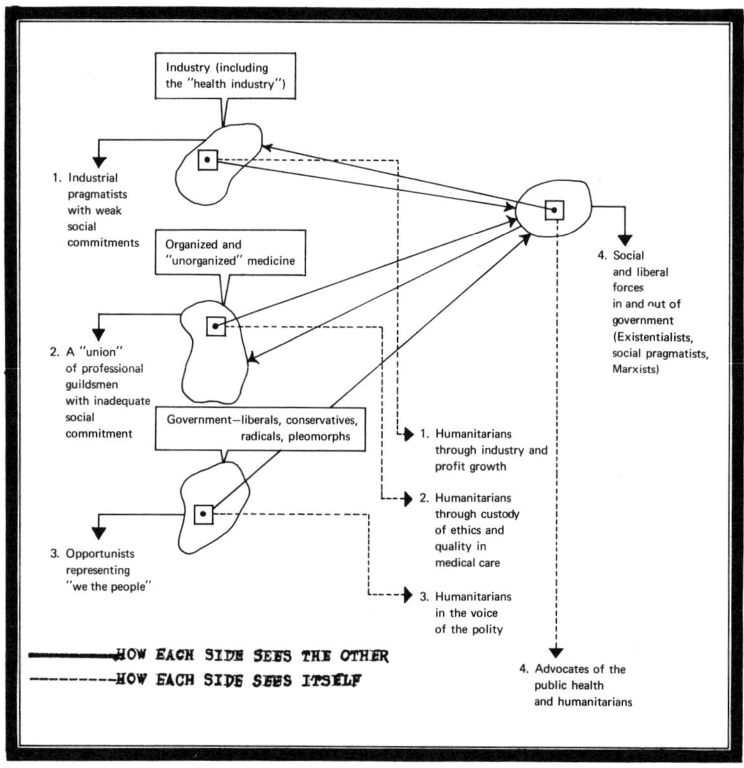

In this exploratory analysis we find the syntheses of opposing views in philosophy and language properly within the purview of the government of the polity, which must decide the "timeliness"*

*It is of interest that 86 years after Bismarck introduced the national health care system in Germany and 58 years after Lloyd George indicated a similar system in England, the timeliness of such systems still remains a matter hotly debated in the U.S.A.

138

of social change, in the light of challenge either in the form of newly discovered techniques or threat of social disaster.

In these decisions the polity's expectations of government can become unrealistic as when the British adopted a "free health service" and expected the service to cost them nothing. All such a health service can be is a form of prepaid medical care where the prepayment is in taxes rather than insurance premiums. Under government taxation, medical care is "free" only in the sense that a profit motive has been removed from its actuarial structure and, by broadening the base of pooling risks, greater protection is available for a greater number of people.* The large numbers of employed persons paying premiums not only to commercial group insurance but to union medical and hospitalization plans would continue to contribute these premiums, but in the form of taxes to a government nonprofit insurance system. Labor would finance the two existing Social Security Systems with employees paying 1 percent of wages up to specified sums, employers and government paying 3 percent from general revenue.

This exploration in awareness has taken us far afield from the central character of this writing, the sick human being. We must be constantly reminded of him in the language interchange of worldly and other philosophies. These philosophies frequently become irrelevant to him in his preoccupation with gaining confidence in those who can cure or favorably modify his affliction. This is

*In any event the author has found the average patient in Britain is happy with this service while there still remains a sizable group of "overworked" physicians who sustain a chronic "unhappiness" with the system (administrative) of medical care. The "evils" of profit motivation become substituted for by the wills of burgeoning administrative superstructures in the delivery of medical care (Parkinson's Law). Presently, England runs a highly technological and interrelated service by means of over 700 individual authorities, three separate types of administrations and two entirely different sources of income (Report of Richard Crossman, Secretary of State for Social Service, in his proposal for reorganization of England's National Health Service). In addition there has been an unplanned growth of private health insurance plans and the more affluent, insured under these plans, are at an advantage in competing for services of physicians and at times scarce hospital beds *(Med. Tribune and Medical News,* Vol. 10, No. 102, December, 1969). What is termed a "blueprint for the future" for Britain's National Health Service proposes a remedial "infusion" of private enterprise in which the illusion of equality in medical care is dispelled. *AMA News* (May 4), 1970.

139

paramount to him when he is sick and hospitalized. It is when he is well and away from hospital care that he begins to ponder the economic "ills" of his past affliction. After leaving the marginal existence of illness he reenters the mainstream of existence as a "refranchised" citizen; he may justifiably ask his friends, the polity, or government why the economic cost of illness is so high.

CHAPTER V

Bergner, L. and Yerby, A. S. "Low Income and Barriers to Use of Health Services." *New England J. Med.*, 278:541-546 (Mar.), 1968.

Breslow, Lester. "The Urgency of Social Action for Health." *Amer. Journal of Public Health,* Vol. 60, No. 1 (Jan.), 1970.

Burns, E. M. "Social Policy and the Health Services: The Choices Ahead." *American Journal of Public Health,* 57:2 (Feb.), 1967.

Burns, E. M. "Some Major Policy Decisions Facing the United States in the Financing and Organization of Health Care." *Bull. New York Acad. Med.,* Second Ser., 42:1072, 1966.

Cohen, W. S. "Current Problems in Health Care." *New England Journal Med.* 281:193-197 (July), 1969.

Cornely, P. B. and Bigman, S. K. *Cultural Considerations in Changing Health Attitudes.* Washington: Howard University, 1961.

Dearing, W. D. "Medicare—Its Meaning to the Consumer." *J. Amer. Geriatrics Soc.,* 14:1087-1094 (Nov.), 1966.

Falk, I. S. "Medical Care and Social Policy." *AJPH,* 55:4:526 (April), 1965.

Fein, O. and C. "Alternatives Facing the Radical in Medicine." Students for a Democratic Society Radical Education Conference, Ann Arbor, Mich., July 1967.

Heilbroner, Robert L. *The Worldly Philosophers.* New York: Simon and Schuster, Inc., 1961.

Hutchins, Robert M. with Lyford, Joseph P. *The Political Animal.* Center for the Study of Democratic Institutions. The Fund for the Republic. Santa Barbara, Calif., 1962.

McNerney, Walter J. *AJPH,* Vol. 59 (Oct.), 1969, 1808.

Medical Association News. Weekly editions (1966-1969).

Medical Care for the American People, XVI, 213 pp. Chicago: University of Chicago Press, 1932.

Medical Care: The Current Scene and Prospects for the Future. Proceedings of Symposium in Honor of I. S. Falk. New Haven: Yale University School of Medicine, May 10-11, 1969 *Journal of Public Health* (Supp.) Vol. 59, No. 1, (Jan.), 1969.

Medical Tribune, (November 20), 1969. A.M.A. Urges Medicredit, Voluntary Health Insurance.

Meissner, H. H. (ed.) *Poverty in the Affluent Society.* New York: Harper & Row, 1966.

Meltsner, M. "Equality and Health." *University of Pennsylvania Law Review,* 115: No. 1 (Nov.), 1966.

141

Miller, S. M. and Riessman, F. *Social Class and Social Policy*. New York: Basic Books, 1968.

Palyi, Melchior. *Compulsory Medical Care and The Welfare State*. Chicago: National Institute of Professional Services, 1949.

Reuther, Walter P. "The Health Care Crisis: Where Do We Go From Here?" *AJPH*, Vol. 59, No. 1 (Jan.), 1969.

Rosen, George in *Handbook of Medical Sociology*. Freeman, H. E.; Levine, S.; and Reeder, I. G. Englewood Cliffs: Prentice-Hall, 1963.

Saunders, L. *Cultural Differences and Medical Care*. New York: Russell Sage Foundation, 1954.

Smith, A. *The Wealth of Nations* (1776). New York: Modern Library, 1937.

Source Book of Health Insurance Data. Health Insurance Institute, New York, 1967.

White, K. L. "Organization and Delivery of Personal Health Services: Public Policy Issues." *Millbank Memorial Fund Quarterly*, 46:225-228 (Jan.), 1968.

Wilson, A. M. "Group Disability Insurance." Paper presented at symposium at Harvard School of Public Health, April 4, 1953. *Ind. Med. and Surgery*, February, 1954.

Winslow, C. E. *The Cost of Sickness and the Price of Health*. Geneva: World Health Organization Monograph Series, 1951.

Woodward, C. "Reality and Social Reform: The Transition From Laissez-Faire to the Welfare State." *Yale Law Journal*, 22, 2:286-328 (Dec.), 1962.

Zsasz, T. S., Kuoff, W. F., and Hollender, M. H. "The Doctor-Patient Relationship In Its Historical Context." *American Journal Psychiat.*, 115:522, 1958.

CHAPTER VI

A Semantic Analysis of Modern Psychiatry

Aside from its jargon or arcanism, from which all specialty language suffers, the verbal "world" of psychiatry is most complex and possesses a host of words lacking common definition or meaning in its nomenclature. Psychiatrists frequently do not agree among themselves on words used to describe diagnosis and disease categories (i.e., autistic, schizophrenic,* manic depressive, *et al.*). As psychiatrists continue to have difficulty with the verbal world physicians, other than psychiatrists, and the public become confused. Verbal problems are related to abstractions of epistomology and of metaphysics. The present crisis in the specialty is similar to those conversations and controversies that occurred among the great philosophers; it has been complicated more recently by influences of more modern analytic and existensial schools of philosophy. As a result psychiatry is forced to review its past, present, and future as a specialty and also its world of words and symbols.

The matrix of psychiatric language reflects upbringing in demonology, theology, the arts, philosophy, literature, and the whole history of man. Psychiatry, historically, shares with the rest of medicine a heritage which at times was monstrous. Physicians and surgeons had their origins in tonsorialism and practices of blood letting, emetics, and purgatives; psychiatrists had theirs in demonology and exorcism. The Ebers Papyrus (c. 1550 B.C.) refers to a period of demonology in Egyptian medicine when all mental illness was considered to be dependent upon evil spirits; thus psychiatry had its earliest language and disease classification within

*For some insight into communication problems among professionals and non-professionals on this subject see: Sankar, Siva, D. U. (ed.) "Schizophrenia: Current Concepts and Research." New York, Hicksville PID Publications, 1970.

the realm of religious and psychological principles. Centuries later these principles remained, with refinements in language. Mental illness was categorized into seven types: five due to the anger of specific evil spirits; one to the anger of gods; one due to the anger of dead men's spirits. These categories presaged Freudian concepts of love and hate drives, guilt fears and phobias. The pendulum of thought on mental illness, however, was swung the other way by Greek writings, which at 500 B.C. conceived it as being due to physiological, organic, or natural causes.

Pythagoras brought mental illness within the realm of a philosophy which placed the intellect in the brain. He considered mental illness therefore a disorder of the brain. Hippocrates propounded theories that conceived of the brain as a gland secreting or excreting substances to all parts of the body. To him the retention of these substances led to mental aberration. As a result he stressed the importance of fresh air to proper function of both blood and brain. As we shall see, Hippocrates' secretory theory in relation to mental illness was to persist until the time of Freud.

In the Middle Ages, there was a reawakening of demonology in psychiatry. Religious dogma had labeled evil spirits within the context of Christian religion; they became known variously as satan, Lucifer, Mephistophales, and the devil. Psychiatry, as a prisoner of religious dogma and witchcraft, was practiced in dungeons and later in places associated with dungeons; then in alms and pest houses, and hell-holes called asylums. Thus the verbal world of psychiatry possessed poor symbolism and arrangement on up to its modern era when psychiatrists, at times, are still referred to as "Alienists."

With the progress made in pathology, physiology, pharmacology, and bacteriology in the eighteenth and nineteenth centuries,* psychiatry again became identified with the organic aspects of medicine. Writers in this period described consciousness as a secretion of the brain in the same sense bile is a secretion of the liver.** As

---

*Freud's initial preoccupation in the field of mental illness was with pharmacology (cocaine) and neuroanatomy and neurophysiology (structure and function of nerve cells).

**Dictum of Cabanis.

in the time of Pythagoras mental illness was explained by organic or structural alteration of the brain. This was a sterile era since psychiatry dealt mainly with mechanistic thinking (based on physiology, physics, and mathematics) with little understanding of meaning of mental symptoms.

It adjusted its language as it looked for principles, seeking them alternately within the realm of physiology and psychology. Meanwhile, through the ages, the truth about the mind or instincts, memory, or consciousness has eluded, to this day, psychiatrists, including Freud, and the great philosophers. All philosophical speculation aside, it is fortunate that most human beings verbally agreed on what they considered to be the mind (as opposed to matter) and were able to communicate to each other generally in terms of its order and disorder. Thus there exists in the verbal world of mental illness one area that is discernable, describable, and possessing a vocabulary: prestigious and utilitarian but which represents only a small part of the total world of events of happenings in psychiatry; the balance remains hidden.

Psychiatry's hidden world faces antimonies in definitions. Its disagreement on terminology in mental illness involves the whole philology: its scope and content. The dissidence becomes broad with general philosophy as the stuff of disparity. An attempt to construct a synthesis in meaning of mental illness even has been postulated on a *mythical* basis. In this destructive 'analysis' of the specialty psychiatry is labeled a 'pseudomedical science' and mental illness pictured as the name given to bias of one group of human beings in describing another.*

In Freud's *Theory of the Mind*, psychiatry discovered what was thought to be its first principles. His psychoanalytic theory, based to a large extent on an intuitive self-analysis, provided a doctrinal

---

*Szasz employs this concept in decrying the continuance of involuntary commitment of "psychiatric" patients to mental institutions. Some of the justification of his thesis may be found in Stuart Mill's Philosophy of Human Rights. This concept makes turnkeys of psychiatrists. A similar view has been operative in society for centuries between the heterosexual and the homosexual; only recently in America have efforts been made to allow freedom to adult homosexuals to be "different" as long as they exercise propriety in not offending sensibilities of those "different" from themselves.

and verbal world, though at times it became the despair of psychiatrists and nonpsychiatrists alike.

Modern psychiatry faces semantic reactions from some quarters of medicine in the form of accusations of cloisterism, indifference, impotence, and failure to move ahead with the rest of medicine. Psychiatrists also have been accused of treating other members of the medical profession as laymen, inferior, and as being unworthy of association.

In isolation from medical colleagues psychiatrists are pictured as unscientific in diagnosis and ineffectual in treatment modalities. The criticism is cloaked in rhethoric: 'medieval attitudes,' 'mystic aloofness,' 'language-locked.' Psychiatry is looked on as a specialty that has turned its back on the *soma* in favor of the *psyche*. There are those in medicine who call psychoanalysis an unscientific 'fad.' Most criticism is leveled at what are termed 'silent Sams' and 'Stonewalls,' the 'listening tapes' whose techniques are nondirective.

Criticism is leveled at psychiatry's nonverbalization of its ideas toward social commitment; as a result there are intimations that it creates economic frames of reference in functioning as a speciality,* helping those who need help least. On matters of social commitment, it appears however that psychiatrists offer no more or no less than their medical colleagues in other branches of medicine. The problem here is that psychiatrists do not live in a common world with other medical practitioners either in daily experience, language, or even philosophy. A philosophy adequate to integrate the world of another medical practitioner may be inadequate in integrating the world of the psychiatrists. Their world views (Weltanschauung) are bound to be different; so too their intensional hidden "unspeakable" worlds may furnish no common outlook on life with the average medical practitioner. What might appear, in the mind of the average medical practitioner, as social

*Psychiatrists often rank in the upper percentile of physicians earning more than $25,000 annually from federally financed medical programs *alone*. (Testimony before Armed Services Comm. on fees paid by the Civilian Health and Medical Programs of the Uniformed Services, Nov. and Dec. 1969).

commitment is easily expressed in the everyday verbal and logical world in terms of service he gives freely to a clinic. This service could represent doctrinal anathema to his psychiatrist counterpart, depending on whether motivations to "donate" such service were due to altruistic love or self-priority.

There is in psychiatry's present semantic relationships with patients a situation different from that of other specialties in the art of healing, in attitudes toward patient criticism, diagnosis, and the psychiatrist's own self-concept in his dialogue with the patient. Both psychiatrist and nonpsychiatrist can to a degree become egotistic and narcissistic. The psychiatrist, however, has learned to be less sure, through training, of his acceptance as an individual by the patient. The nonpsychiatrist is surprised when the patient is unyielding or critical; he feels threatened and may react defensively either in mood or manner. The psychiatrist deals with criticism or rejection objectively and often in a constructive and eventually therapeutic manner. Nonpsychiatrists seek a *static* label to place on the patient's condition, such as acute, subacute, chronic, or progressive. Having ruled out organic disease with reasonable certainty psychiatrists become concerned with a *dynamic* formulation, where the patient may not be the same person on succeeding visits to their offices.

Principles of language and philosophy discussed elsewhere in this book often do not apply to the patient-physician relationship in the diagnosis and treatment of mental illness. Empathetic principles involving language of *caritas*, which should usually take place in the personal interchange between physician and patient, are not usual in psychiatry. In fact "Stonewall" responses, language barriers, or semantic deadlocks may be used by the psychiatrist to help construct a therapeutic relationship. He may consider language of support and reassurance a proper tool in specific instances but improper as a basic professional attitude because in instances it proves a diagnostic and therapeutic barrier. It is no wonder, in the verbal world, that psychiatry at times has been considered cloistered, aloof, asocial, since such guarded speech, lacking emotional tone, is heard not only by patients but by colleagues in other specialties.

147

The rest of medical practice has only within a decade or two come under criticism for its impersonal mode of dealing with patients; psychiatry has for a half-century considered detachment (the "Alienist") part of the specialty. It has placed great emphasis on patient volition, a free-flowing relationship. At times even suicides remain unknown to attending psychiatrists for extended periods after their patient's death. Within frames of reference in other aspects of medical practice this situation could fall within the realm of patient abandonment.

Much of psychiatry's image has been created by perplexities in acceptance of the validity of psychological data. Physicians accustomed to objective observed data on physical conditions frequently brush aside psychological data because of its intangibility; this condition will remain as long as psychology and the humanities remain deficient in medical curricula.

It is on the validity of psychological theory that most language in conceptualization of personality is based. Here, at times, psychiatry's *intensional* world (word) often is at odds with the *extensional* world (experience) of other members of the healing art, who consider their own work to be primarily scientific and objective. If their verbal world had through education been conditioned to psychoanalytic theory, perhaps other physicians would view or experience the human personality in a way more parallel to the psychiatrist's. Upon this merging of awareness depends the mutual understanding of psychiatrist by nonpsychiatrist and also survival of holistic concepts in human beings.* In holistic concepts, language of physical, chemical, psychological, and sociological influences becomes equally relevant in identifying or explaining mental disorder. This is quite comprehensive and different from diagnosing a broken bone.

Stemming from Freudian thinking is the theoretical concept of personality anatomy where "pathology" of mental disease is postulated into the world of symbols in the familiar diagram:

---

*It is of interest that in some countries, such as the Republic of Ireland, as much as 90 percent of mental or emotional problems of patients are treated by nonpsychiatrists.

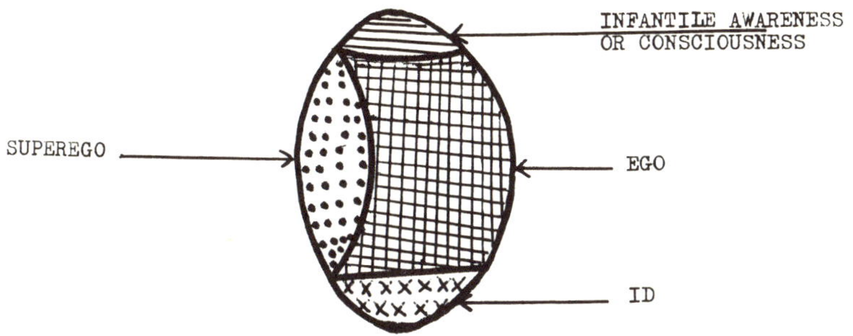

This diagram unfortunately became the symbolic language of the whole "mechanism" of personality. Those accustomed, by training, to speculative deductions, relating to unknown factors, found the model a useful explanation of personality and its functions and disorders. It enabled them to coordinate and compare experiences with others within some useful framework of reference. This model had legitimacy as a theoretical concept of personality anatomy and reduced appreciably barriers and complexities in language when psychiatrists compare, in the verbal world, their experiences and happenings in diagnosing and treating mental illness. While this word world of the personality generally is useful, it represents oversimplification of events and forces at work in the hidden world of human personality.

Psychiatric language puts much emphasis on the feelings of those working with troubled personalities and on how they feel toward the psychiatrists. While striving for objectivity in this relationship, psychiatrists do not escape spontaneous communicative deadlocks (conflict of "worlds") in unavoidable exchange of feelings, which affect both patient and psychiatrist. These feelings influence therapy and the foundation of therapeutic relationships. Psychiatrists have placed great importance upon "blind spots" and their own personality deviation in listening and communicating with troubled human beings. This is most difficult since there is very little overlapping of the common world, especially of a physician, and the average patient (based on dissimilarity of experience, culture, and language).

It was not until the turn of the twentieth century and the advent of Freud (a man of letters *par excellence*) that psychiatry's verbal and doctrinal worlds returned to psychical processes,* a language that led to better understanding of symptoms in mental disorders. Whether or not one wishes to accept validity of Freudian analysis or to accept Freud is of little importance in light of the incontrovertible fact that he gave psychiatry (as a result of his self-analysis) a useful theory of human behavior and a language having doctrinal relationships and propositions related to the verbal world of philosophy, literature, drama, history, and the arts. Not only has psychiatry become literature; at times literature becomes psychiatry.** Freud's case histories *(Dora)* had real characters in the sense of a novel or play. Freud already has caused alterations in how history, news, plays, and novels are written. We see Freud's concept of interior consciousness displayed in Joyce and Woolf or by television writers, in nonlinear efforts to reach beyond the narrative form.

These and other considerations indicate that psychiatry past and present has been a precocious child of medicine, mainly because during history its silent, unspeakable, mysterious regions of events presented doctrinal complexities, difficult to express in the common language and logic of words and symbols.

Misinformation bred in a vacuum created by psychiatry's isolation and lack of communication led many in and out of the profession to ask the question, "Is the psychoanalyst a physician," thinking, "If he is, he ought to 'behave' like one; if he is not, he

---

*Freud became convinced that psychical processes should be treated in language of psychological not physiological data; physiological data already had become too closely harmonized with the language of physics and chemistry.

**Thomas Mann once remarked he deplored all the hard work Freud had undergone in his scientific investigation, a labor from which he could have been spared by greater pursuit of knowledge of literature.

should not use the title 'M.D.' to add prestige to his methods."* These thoughts are mainly those of activist physicians, who question any emphasis on theory rather than direct therapy.

Psychoanalysis has become a whipping boy and partially displaced by behavior or conditioning therapy; this is testimony not so much to its inadequacies as a theory but to default on the part of psychiatrists in communicating its principles and doctrines. Intramural dissension among Freudian analysts on points of *theory* was translated by the medical profession generally and the public as disputation on points of *fact*. Also, while analysts agreed to disagree on theory, they forgot they were dealing with theory to begin with.** In other fields (say, nuclear physics) the disagreement on theories usually is maintained within confines of academic enclosures (partially hidden world) with barriers to widespread publicity.

Psychiatry has learned important lessons in semantic analysis and in the verbalization of any particular doctrinal theory or propositional dogma in treatment of mental illness. There remain however large numbers of psychoanalysts and practitioners trained or influenced by analysts, whose therapeutic approach continues to be entirely psychological and nondirective. Emphasis is on gaining and application of insight (in the patient). This group (A-P) performs no physical examinations or prescribes any drugs or organic treatment. Also there are many practitioners with different approaches to therapy who believe in changing patients' attitudes and behavior by directive methods (suggestion, reassurance, and

*Some of this attitude (mainly erroneous) stems historically from aspects of cultism found among the early membership of the International Psychoanalytical Association (c. 1910-'14). Freud believed that inevitable and considerable opposition to his psychoanalytic theory would stem from Anti-Semitism as it did in the schism between the Viennese (mainly Jewish) and Swiss (mainly Christian) groups of psychoanalysts. Also promulgation of "lay analysis" in the Association caused divisive opinion and their open conflict spurred lay and professional attacks on psychoanalysis and its practitioners.

**Dissension over theory in psychological data occurred early among original members of the International Psychoanalytical Association (Ferenczi versus Viennese group; Bleuler versus Jung; Bleuler versus Freud; Abraham versus Jung; Freud versus Adler).

151

reproof) and who prescribe drugs, medical or neurological examinations as necessity demands.

Through thesis and antithesis, combinations of psychoanalytic and behavioristic approaches are being used with broad frameworks of psychotherapeutic regimens; whether the behaviorists will win out remains problematical. History of the specialty teaches that where there has been "overinvestment" in treatment methods there will also be found rigid dogma.

Particularly disturbing to the public are those statistics on therapeutic results indicating adverse effects of psychoanalysis and psychotherapy on individual chances for recovery. Some of these statistics indicate: better therapeutic results without any treatment; the results of trained psychiatrists less successful than those of social workers and psychologists; and results of untrained aides better than both groups of trained professionals. Reflecting some bias in case selection, these statistics would indicate an inverse ratio existing between schooling or training and therapeutic sophistication. These statistics indicate that in the art of medicine, interpersonal relationships of trust, confidence, sensitivity, and empathy are derivatives not of educational systems but of personal attributes of the individuals involved in the relationship. They infer also that a large percentage of mental illness may be approached therapeutically through bonds of empathy among patients' family, friends, relatives, fellow employees, or other members of their community; perhaps persons able to solve their mental problems in this manner should do so, rather than take some of the calculated risks of formal psychiatric care.

When much of psychiatry turned to Freud and psychoanalysis three quarters of a century ago, the family and other potentially empathetic groups became part of the hidden world of happenings and events for both patient and practitioner. The language or communications world for the patient frequently changed from his intimates to a "closed" relationship with the therapist who was to become *his* true friend, *his* confidant and supporter, in the patient's conflicts with the "outside" world. Where vacuums of information are created, families and friends react semantically with misunderstanding, feel rebuffed, and are sometimes infuriated. Family physicians and families who receive no progress reports feel alienated, giving meaning to the title "Alienist,"* other than the usually accepted meaning of the word among psychiatrists. Therapists frequently fail to explain to families the need to identify with the patient's "cause" against the outside world. Also unexplained to intimates of the patient is the therapist's fear that listening to them would weaken his relationship with the patient.

Thus we see a therapeutic modality, based on Freudian theory of the mind, causing semantic reactions beyond the one-to-one relationship of patient and therapist. A modality that can isolate the patient's word world from that of his family and other intimates was bound to have repercussions, generally, in the public's attitudes toward psychiatry's commitment or lack of it to the social order.

When the specialty later refocused attention on the patient's family, social groups, and communities and positive mental health, there was a change in its verbal world; this was true especially among therapists working in neighborhood clinics. In dealing with social and cultural factors of mental illness in individual patients close to their environs, therapists became increasingly aware of mental disorder in terms of multiple personal and environmental rather than one-to-one relationships. Lines of communications were opened between the therapist, his patient, and the patient's medical practitioner; his family, friends, and relatives.** The

*During the first third of this century, the consultant in psychiatry was called an alienist and his work related only casually to the practice of medicine. The demand for diagnosis and treatment of mental disorders increased and soon every psychiatrist, even those in fledgling years of training, became consultants to the medical profession. Unfortunately, as already has been indicated, there were barriers in communication between psychiatrists and nonpsychiatrists. The languages of medical pathology and psychopathology differed. The metaphysical inspirations of Freud and neopsychoanalytic concepts dominated teaching in many medical schools. This in most instances confused rather than enlightened the nonpsychiatrist. (See Commes, Leonard. "From Alienist to Consultant." *Medical Opinion and Review,* Vol. 5, No. 12 (December), 1969.

**Many psychiatrists of this present decade have diminished their authoritarian symbolism and have realistically reexamined their contribution to positive health maintenance of patients. Thus many are returning to the mainstream of medicine and have learned to integrate their efforts into understandable and believable language in total patient care.

"silent" world of events and happenings in mental illness changed as well as its symbols, "logic," and words.

In this approach intimates of patients gain better understanding of themselves, which often benefits the patient. The patient understands more clearly how his language and actions affect intimates and they in turn see how their language and actions affect the patient. Within these areas of understanding in language and action are those factors that frequently govern relapses or continued progress among patients who are discharged back to homes and jobs free of hallucinations, fears, phobias, or mental symptoms generally.

In areas of positive mental health, the language of psychiatry is changing along with society, so that as a specialty it can assist in diagnosing and treating cultural illness and social disorder. There is greater interest shown by psychiatrists in sociological and anthropological concepts of mental disease in relationship to static (primitive) and dynamic societies such as we live in today.

In brief, modern psychiatry has learned that it cannot operate as a specialty in a vacuum devoid of communications in the verbal world of social values and doctrines. To promote research and clinical practice, it cannot isolate itself from the social scientist or from the rest of the medical profession. If psychiatry looks to its future realistically it will find itself heavily involved not only in prevention of mental illness but in semantics, which will become increasingly important in educating the public in the meaning and causes of mental disorders. The future of research and prevention in mental illness will be measurable in terms of whether practice of psychiatry will require in the future an increased or lessened reliance on drugs or the evolution of psychopharmacology.

To date, drug treatment of patients* has been regarded with ambivalence by psychiatrists and there has been a lag or gap in knowledge and language created by a rapid evolution of pharmacology in relation to a slower, almost static, evolution of psy-

---

*Freud, early in his career, considered cocaine somewhat of a "miracle" drug and became much preoccupied with its pharmacological and therapeutic effects, which he tested on himself and his friends.

chodynamics. The modern era of pharmacology, in which as many as 70 percent of patients are treated with medications either as a substitute or adjunct to psychotherapy, attests to the fact that use of psychotropic drugs is outpacing psychodynamic principles in the approach to cause and treatment of mental illness. This predicament is indicative of another cyclic phase in the history of psychiatry (as in the time of Pythagoras and Hippocrates) where physiological principles have ascendency over psychological ones. To harmonize these principles (in psychiatry's hidden world) requires revision of psychiatric theory, practice, education, and the equally herculean task of harmonizing the tendencies of biological, physiological, and psychological data—a task Freud feverishly attempted without success.

When we speak of a physiological or biological tendency in psychiatry we find the specialty lacking words and symbols as found in the objective observations or measurements of physiology or biology. There is no language in psychiatry comparable to "blood sugar" and "glucose tolerance" tests used in internal or general medicine. Thus while the psychiatrist may deal with approaches to diagnoses and treatment of a psychobiological nature, his evaluations or measurement of efficacy in these approaches remain within the sphere of psychology and psychodynamics; these approaches are mainly located in the psychiatrist's own world of events, happenings, propositions, and doctrines.

In other words, lacking precise or objective biochemical or physiological measurements, psychiatry continues to rely upon judgments in evaluations coming from within the observer. These evaluations are affected by a wide variety of factors: the clinician's own motivations (conscious or unconscious); his skepticism or rather bias on efficacy of drug therapy; his "response set" in evaluating; his "halo" world, which rates particulars on the basis of generalities (doctrinal and propositional).

To complicate evaluations in drug therapy are variables in the patient's private world affecting his verbal report: his attitude and feelings (religious, etc.) and past history regarding the taking of drugs; the patient's attitude toward intimates or others in his life he associates with taking drugs; his response to change in contact

with reality brought on by medication; his articulateness in report-
ing effects of drugs; and impressions gained from other patients
using the same drug. Added problems are the symbols of different
environmental influences contained in the setting of drug therapy:
the nature of the institution (voluntary or involuntary commitment,
locked or unlocked wards, etc.); the degree of crowding; and
the state of harmony or disharmony in the therapeutic setting.

Therefore, in attempts to harmonize the psychological language
of psychiatry with physiology and pharmacology, there are complex interacting variables. Since objective judgment of the interaction of these variables is markedly limited at present their
assessment becomes a subjective measurement of symptom change
with no "unified" approach in language to bridge strictly psychological, pharmacological, and physiological theory. All present
theories remain provisional for want of a unified theory for cause,
prevention, or treatment of mental illness. Thus there appears a
need, in psychiatry's hidden doctrinal world (unspeakable), for
linking psychodynamic and psychobiological theory.* In its
research, education, and practice, this linking would furnish
psychiatry a "speakable" world of happenings, of what is going
on in the specialty; this in turn would cause a greater degree of

*Freud hoped, in promoting lay analysis, for the spread and integra-
tion of psychoanalytic theory into disciplines other than medicine; i.e.,
biological science generally; anthropology; sociology; history, including
religious history. Some of his hopes had borne fruit during his lifetime.
After his death, Freudian theory too slowly sought expression of usefulness outside the confines of mental illness. One notable exception to
this was Alexander Leighton's work in the Poston Relocation Camp
during World War II, where he applied his training in psychiatry and
anthropology to social and other problems arising among the Japanese
relocated in this desolate area of Arizona. Later Erik Erikson in the
writing of his book, "Young Man Luther" in an excellent fashion exem-
plified integration of psychoanalysis with religious history. See Erikson,
Erik H. *Young Man Luther—A Study in Psychoanalysis and History*. New
York: W. W. Norton & Co., Inc. 1962.

Franz Alexander, who attempted integration of Freudian analytical
insights with those of "organic medicine" emphasized that psychoanalysis
had done its share as "an operational psychological tool." He repeatedly
expressed in his writings "the need for coordination of psychoanalytic
findings (principles) with physiology and the social sciences." (See Alexander, Franz: *The Western Mind in Transition*. New York: Random
House, pp. 57-62; 62-66, 1960). His emphasis on organ vulnerability in
psychosomatics had added implications of a "disease choice" by indi-

common awareness in the verbal worlds among psychiatrists, other practitioners of the healing art, and the public.

Adding urgency to attempts at harmonizing sociologic, psychodynamic and psychobiological or pharmacologic tendencies in psychiatry is man's urge for self-transcendence, made more compelling by his modern imprisonment in a social and economic system of his own invention.

There exists in all human beings a universal proclivity toward self-transcendence. (Every time I look at me I only see me in me; oh Lord! let me see other than me in me.) While man always wished to escape imprisonment of himself and his personality, today he has greater desire than ever for escape to a less painful reality of himself and his modern existence. The religious attribute this desire for self-transcendence to an innate deep-seated yearning for the divine. Biologists see it as a working of man's innate gregariousness. The individual frequently sees this tendency in the light of his own self-centeredness; he longs to be merged with the herd but feels too self-conscious or is too egocentric to sustain the merging effort very long. Modern man therefore finds himself, like his ancestors, condemned to live in a state of chronic dissatisfaction, pining for things he can never have. Historically man has "solved" his dissatisfied feelings by chemical methods, musical or gymnastic methods, methods depending upon subjection to influences of crowds (herd poisoning), and those of

viduals. This perhaps was the greatest onslaught upon the cause- and-effect mechanistic dogmas (Freud shared in these) of medicine, held inviolate since Virchow, Welch, and Osler. These dogmas became even more vulnerable in light of the work of Cannon and later Hans Selye in the field of organism stress.

Today there is a large body of evidence supporting endocrine, chemical (serotinin, abnormal adrenalin, lithium and magnesium salts) of mental diseases such as schizophrenia (para-phrenia) and cyclothymia (manic-depressive disease). The postulation of chemical theory, which would bridge the work of Freud, Alexander, Cannon, and Selye becomes an interesting speculation for inclusion within the doctrinal world of psychiatry. The author feels obliged to add the anthropologic studies of Alexander Leighton as a condition of fulfilling Franz Alexander's plea to coordinate psychoanalytic theory with physiology and social sciences.

Still we must deal in semantic context, with Szasz's postulation of mental illness on a "mythical" basis, which pictures the bias of groups in society toward "different" members of society and the effects of this bias on basic human rights.

157

mysticism, religion, and spiritual exercises of Oriental or Western tradition. He has found in these methods changes in consciousness giving him a degree of self-transcendence and relief from his tension of discontent.

Chemical compounds whether in root, twig, leaf, flower, seed, or ferment provided man, even in paleolithic times, with a measure of self-transcendence and relief. While adding genius of synthesis and extraction, modern pharmacology in its psychobiological approach has added nothing to man's art of proclivity in seeking surcease through natural remedies in his environment. Most naturally occurring sedatives, narcotics, euphorics, and combinations thereof were discovered thousands of years ago, before the dawn of civilization. In his organic evolution man employed these first to poison his enemies and by the late Stone Age to poison himself. The presence of poppy heads in the kitchen middens of Swiss Lake Dwellers attests to man's early discovery of techniques for self-poisoning in his effort to discover techniques in self-transcendence. These techniques discovered prior to the agricultural age of man indicate he was a drug addict before becoming a farmer.*

Historically man judged as "good" anything that produced self-transcendence regardless of long-term consequences. Tribal and cultural "medications" whether they are the peyote of the Navaho, the opium hashish of Islam, the *soma* of India, the wine of Israel, or the mead of the Anglo-Saxon have been bound with man's need to stimulate his mystical faculties. This need has existed regardless of man's religious state, although transcendence produced by tribal and cultural medication was often identified with one or another god.

Semantically the ecstatic release took on such a large connotation of the supernatural that these mental states, according to effects, became personalized and named as deities and pagan gods. Wine to the Greeks was not merely sacred to Dionysus; wine *was* Dionysus. Bacchus was called *theoinos*—Godwine—a single word equating alcohol with deity. The word opium had been

*Aldous Huxley. "The History of Tension." *Annals of New York Academy of Sciences,* Vol. 67, Art. 10, pp. 671-894.

equated with the word *religion* among far-Eastern and Asiatic tribes long before Marx metaphorically called *religion* the opium of the people. In ancient India the *soma* plant was not merely sacred to the hero god Indra; the soma *was* Indra. Nordic barbarian tribes worshiped beer under the name of Sabazius; beer was the god of the Celts, Scandinavians, Teutons. Anglo-Saxon words meaning catastrophe, panic, ultimate in horror and disaster derive their meaning from "the deprivation of mead." The Indians of the southwestern United States still identify the peyote cactus with native deities and with the Holy Spirit of Christian theology.

Where there are prohibitions, religious or otherwise, in the use of tribal or cultural medications, substitute means are sought to satisfy urges within a culture for self-transcendence. While alcohol is forbidden in the orthodox Moslem world, *cannabis indica* (hashish or marijuana) becomes not only sanctioned by its society but used as a religious rite. Tobacco along with alcohol became cultural medications mainly of the western world.* As these drugs meet greater proscriptions by society they will be substituted for by medications that could be either more or less hazardous to human health.

While Greeks thought men perceived and received "good" from Bacchus, attempts among the Jews to give drink complete religious sanction were thwarted by various priests and prophets. Beyond the wedding cup and the "cup of consolation" referred to by Jeremiah we have harsh words for the use of alcohol by Mica and by Isaiah, who denounced priests and prophets who erred "in vision" through strong drink.

In addition to tribal and cultural medications and to religion, man has attained degrees of self-transcendence through strictly social means. Man has been able to intoxicate himself through devotion to familial, professional, or other groups and simply by being a member of a crowd. Though his group participations are apt to be structured and purposeful his crowd activities at times, though self-emerging, become chaotic. He can become unreasoned,

---

*While proscriptions against use of tobacco gain momentum in western cultures, attitudes of health and law enforcement agencies have become more liberal toward possession and use of marijuana.

unmoral—and suddenly, as if poisoned by a drug. This herd poisoning or crowd intoxication becomes self-transcendence of the type sought by the bored indolent citizenry of Rome in circuses and amphitheaters.

All previous means mentioned used by man to change the quality of his consciousness seem surpassed by the advent of psychobiology and psychopharmacology. Pharmacologists hold promise of giving most human beings many self-transcendents, which would provide joy, peace, and loving kindness. These would surpass the effects of the "ancient" drugs, alcohol, or opiates in providing changes in consciousness without exacting the high price men have to pay in resorting to the use of the ancient drugs. Some sociologists predict there will be a massive need for new cultural medications to cure the unhappiness of large numbers of persons who will become lost (except to self-awareness) and powerless in ever growing complexities of modern society. These will be mainly the nonpoor who become unwilling or unable to use social or spiritual means of self-transcendence and the poor who have no great dedication to struggle for a purpose or to become transcended through the herd poisoning of the crowd.

Persons lost in complexities of society and lacking human connections will lack also what the Greeks termed *dialectos* (discussion, debate, argument, conversation, or just plain talk). They will require cultural medications in proportion to degrees to which they become insulated or isolated from these and other communal satisfactions, regardless of their economic status.

The emergency treatment of this lack in self-transcendence in large population groups will be "symptomatic" and pharmacologic well in advance of possible preventive measures based either on psychodynamics or sociology. Whether this emergency treatment produced by pharmacologic evolution or revolution will be considered "good" or "bad" depends upon usefulness of alternatives whether in the form of spiritual exercises or in the restructuring of social, political, economic and physical environments.

Long before psychiatry has reconciled its psychodynamic principles and language with psychobiological principles it may be called upon to shoulder the unfair burden of diagnosis and treatment of a cultural sickness based on social factors. While presently the specialty may lack language or skill for this task, the task is relevant to psychological principles and belongs to psychiatry as well as other disciplines. Perhaps harmonizing psychodynamic principles with those of cultural, social, and political forces may be more urgent than coming to grips with the evolution in psychopharmacology or psychobiology. Then psychiatry with propriety can accept the challenge to actualize man's potential to become the best of all animals (hominization). In harmonizing its psychodynamic tendencies and language with problems of widespread sickness in the social and cultural order, psychiatry can assist in structuring a therapeutic (love bond) society. This society would be the ultimate in evolution of the psychosocial order (the noosphere). Failure of forces to structure a therapeutic society will be measurable in the predominance of psychopharmacology over all other modalities of psychiatry. Human beings on a massive scale will then resort to cultural medications with or without religiousness in order to escape imprisonment of their own personalities, to seek joy, peace, and loving kindness and still moments of reflection and contemplation. Temporarily evolutionary trends toward unification of the psychosocial order and toward a hyperpersonal organization of man may be guided by chemicals rather than "natural" cultural or social evolution.

CHAPTER VI

Alexander, Franz. *Psychosomatic Medicine.* New York: W. W. Norton & Co., Inc., 1950.

Blake, Robert R. and Ramsey, Glenn V. (eds.). *Perception, An Approach to Personality.* New York: The Ronald Press, 1951.

Brown, J. A. C. *Techniques of Persuasion.* London: Penguin, 1964, Chapter 8.

Cohen, Sidney. *The Beyond Within.* New York: Atheneum, 1964, Chapter 11.

Freud, Sigmund. *Dora—An Analysis of a Case of Hysteria.* New York: Basic Books, 1963.

Haley, Jay. "The Art of Psychoanalysis" in *The Use and Misuses of Language*, S. I. Hayakawa (ed.). Greenwich: Fawcett Publications, Inc., 1962.

Huxley, Aldous. *Brave New World Revisited.* New York: Bantam Books, 1960, Chapter VIII.

Huxley, Aldous. "Culture and the Individual." In *LSD: Consciousness-Expanding Drug*, David Solomon (ed.). New York: Putnam, 1964, p. 316.

Huxley, Aldous. "Drugs That Shape Men's Minds" in *Adventures of the Mind*, Richard Thruelsen *et al.* (eds.). New York: Alfred A. Knopf, 1959, pp. 90-91.

Huxley, Aldous. *Heaven and Hell.* New York: Harper & Row, 1963, p. 85.

Huxley, Aldous. *The Doors of Perception.* New York: Harper & Row, 1963, p. 40.

Huxley, Aldous. *The Doors of Perception* and *Heaven and Hell.* Baltimore: Penguin Books, 1959, p. 22.

Huxley, Aldous. "The History of Tension." *Annals of New York Academy of Sciences*, Vol. 67, Art. 10, pp. 671-894.

Jahoda, M. *Current Concepts of Positive Mental Health.* New York: Basic Books, 1958.

Johnson *et al. Comprehensive Psychiatry.* 9:563, 1968.

Jones, Ernest, *The Life and Work of Sigmund Freud.* Vols. I, II and III. New York: Basic Books, Inc., 1959.

Leighton, Alexander. The Poston experiment and more recent studies in Newfoundland.

Leighton, A. H. *My Name Is Legion.* New York: Basic Books, Inc. 1959.

May, Jacques M. *A Physician Looks at Psychiatry.* New York: John Day Co., 1958.

McCord, Cary P. "Bloodletting and Bandaging—Barber Surgery as an Occupation. *Arch. Environ. Health,* Vol. 20 (April), 1970.

Menninger Clinic Seminars, Menninger Clinic, Topeka, Kansas (1962).

Moore, Burgess E.; Fine, Bernard D. *A Glossary of Psychoanalytic Terms and Concepts.* New York: American Psychoanalytic Assoc., 1969.

Mullahy, Patrick (ed.). *A Study of Interpersonal Relations.* New York: Hermitage Press Inc., 1949.

Peek, H. "Some Relationships Between Group Process and Mental Health Phenomena in Theory and Practice." *International Journal of Group Psychotherapy,* 13: 3, 1963.

Reissman, F. and Rein, M. "Social Change Versus the Psychiatric World View." *American Journal of Orthopsychiatry,* XXIV:29-38 (Jan.), 1964.

Roesch, Jurgen and Bateson, Gregory. *Communication, the Social Matrix of Psychiatry.* New York: W. W. Norton & Co. Inc., 1951.

Rose, Arnold M. (ed.). *Mental Health and Mental Disorder—A Sociological Approach.* New York: W. W. Norton & Co., Inc., 1955.

Schofield, William. *The Purchase of Friendship.* New York: Prentice-Hall, 1964.

Schwab, John J. *Handbook of Psychiatric Consultation.* New York: Appleton-Century-Crofts.

Sullivan, Harry Stack. *The Psychiatric Interview.* New York: W. W. Norton & Co., Inc., 1954.

Szasz, T. S. Myth of Mental Illness, Foundations of a Theory of Personal Conduct. New York: Harper, 1961.

Woolley, D. W. "The Revolution in Pharmacology" in *Life and Disease,* Dwight J. Ingle (ed.). New York: Basic Books, 1963.

Young, S. *Annals of the Barber-Surgeons.* London: Blades, East & J. Blades, 1890.

CHAPTER VII

Paths Ahead for the Healing Art

If we seek paths ahead for the healing art we must look beyond imminent partial conquests of infectious, degenerative, and malignant disease;* beyond problems, economic and otherwise, in delivery of quality medical care; and to imminent environmental, ecologic, and ekistic** problems. As we study the modern world we can project future developments for which man is responsible and which will occur at the expense of man.

We mentioned earlier that man's organic or biologic evolution was not over; heretofore he had responded fairly successfully, during the evolutionary process, in creating both problems and their solutions in adapting to his external and internal environments. This "leisurely" process of adaptation, spread over millions of years, gave man time, genetically, to achieve a degree of biological equilibrium or homeostasis so that a proportion of the human race has been able to survive threats coming from within its internal environment and from stressful or hostile forces in the

*Forecasts for the future of the healing art follow lines of awareness—surgeons predict better methods of tissue matching between donors and recipients; internists predict solution of terminal kidney disease and methods of controlling arterosclerosis; improvement in scope and quality of medical care with use of computers; yet hopefully with more concern for social and psychologic aspects of disease.

**The science of human settlements.

external world. In fact man's survival, in such great numbers, has caused great concern as a problem in sociology and environmental health.* Suddenly, within the past twenty or thirty years, the upsurge in man's numbers, inventiveness, industry, and discovery poses threats, timewise, to his relatively slow evolution in adaptive capacity. These threats, being biophysical (environmental contamination, radioactive and otherwise) and sociocultural (population explosion and implosion, etc.), affect the health— disease—death continuum of man.** As long as man's ego or his instinct for self-preservation survives, he will remain the center of

*While in the past, the great proportion of modern man's energy, time, and money spent in population studies related to business forecasts for marketable goods, now, mainly through private foundations and centers for study of population growth, energy, time and much money are spent in solving problems of population explosion and implosion, listed by many in polity science and government as "the number one health problem." The findings of these studies have propelled physicians, sociologists, politicians, *et al.* into pressuring law makers in liberalization of birth control laws and regulations (relating to "criminal" abortion); in some instances, the hithertofore "bad man," the abortionist, takes on heroic qualities. It appears, in all of the discussions of population growth, the professionals and the laity have discounted possibilities of cataclysmic events, either "natural" or man made, that will radically change the forecast for future human population growth. Today no right-thinking geneticist or biomedical scientist would venture a prediction as to what the "optimum" population of the world should be. Nor would there be lasting validity to any such figure in view of the dynamics of human organic and social evolution.

We find the healing art entering its initial phase in "exterminative medicine," which as described (mainly by Roman Catholic hierarchy) is a final solution to wiping out the poor and hungry of much of the world's problems in welfare and favors the more affluent who share greater responsibility in environmental problems of the world.

The author does not feel it appropriate in this writing to discuss conflicting philosophies and theories about individualization of the human fetus as a link in the species. He is concerned however about unnatural affects of a broken "lovebond" between mother and fetus, a bond which could be established even under the most adverse social and psysiologic circumstances in pregnancy. The likelihood of lifetime persistency of unconscious maternal mourning must be considered by those who strongly advocate "exterminative medicine."

Should more widespread surgical intervention occur, larger numbers of persons in our society with varying degrees of anxiety or depression could also occur. Those planning for surgical intervention of pregnancy must also plan for larger facilities for the mentally disturbed.

**Depending upon the degree of industrialization and population growth in emerging nations, the world could pollute itself out of existence in from thirty to fifty years.

concern in threats emanating from his environment, both sociological and biological. Ecology* until now has not been seriously considered to be within the purview of the healing art; neither can it hold in the future all the solutions to the health problems of man. Its application to human circumstances, however, is unavoidable now and in the future to preventive medicine, as part of an interdisciplinary approach to those biological and social problems created by man's own inventiveness. It represents potentially another disciplinary reinforcement in medicine's area of greatest need: the holistic approach to man's present and future problems in man's health—disease—death spectrum.

In matters of health, disease, and death we cannot separate human ecology from what Doxiadis termed *ekistics*. Doxiadis states "modern technology has the power to bring men together —but it can also separate them with unforeseen barriers."** He states further that "Everyone must be given the maximum number of choices in order to create his own way of living in all scales, at all community levels. This is society's greatest responsibility toward the individual—not to decrease his choices by arbitrary judgments and decisions on the 'shrinking earth' but to increase all his chances to choose among all scales, at all levels, for all qualities and ages."*** Doxiadis' observations have great meaning and cogency as we look toward paths ahead for the healing art, both for the twentieth-century man and for his descendants.

Future ecologic and ekistic problems of man, the burden of which contemporary medicine must share with engineering and

*The ecologist conceives the term "conservation" as the wise management and utilization of natural resources for the greatest good of the largest number. One may debate the position of man in such a universe, but only as to what level of hierarchy he may allocate himself. That he exists and affects his own kind and all else in the world is not debatable . . . man's history justifies the claim that he, like most other animal and plant life, is "an endangered species." . . . Man, in his struggle for survival, poses as many true ecological challenges as the more familiar lion, rhinocerous, or whooping crane. The environment truly may be his friend or enemy. (See transactions, World Health Organization—Medical Ecology, Geneva, 1969.)

**"Man and the Space Around Him," C. A. Doxiadis, *Saturday Review,* (December 14), 1968.

***Ibid.

the natural, physical, and social sciences, will require further harmonization of medical principles and language with these disciplines. As a result the verbal world of public health specialists may become indistinguishable from that of engineers and physical and social scientists. This will isolate the specialty of public health even more from individual relationships with human beings found in other branches of contemporary medicine; and bring it even closer to the drafting-board approach in solution of problems in the health—disease—death continuum of man.

Man of the twentieth century, so we find, has, through discovery, awakened to more frightening horizons than his forefathers ever knew (nuclear energy excluded). What disconcerts modern human beings most is uncertainty over a *suitable* outcome to discovery of knowledge and uncertainty of individuals as to their proper place among millions of other human beings. Human beings through their own means have become afflicted by the maladies of immensity, complexity, multitude, and uncertainty.

The dilemma of modern discovery is that on one hand it affords the human race, externally, a superior form of existence; and on the other, evolution has not carried the human race beyond its "organic" crises to a psychosocial order in which man is prepared to walk in the direction of his discovery with absolute optimism. Yet there seems to be no middle path in human progress —between attitudes of absolute optimism and absolute pessimism; the polity usually provides no archaistic formulas either to reverse or overthrow progress.

What we term technological progress today is not as old as the first stone axe fashioned by cavemen or as old as the invention of the wheel, the lever, or the cotton gin, or even the assembly line. The "progress" Adam Smith spoke of in *The Wealth of Nations* and the "progress" spoken of in modern times by Orwell and Aldous Huxley do not have the same semantic connotation. The machinery of the first industrial revolution mainly served man, though there were concomitant social and medical problems in the transition from cottage to factory systems of manufacture. Undoubtedly to the mind of the nineteenth and early twentieth centuries, mass production under factory systems appeared an equally sweeping change as modern automatic methods of production do today. The significant difference between the two types of progress in industrial production has proven to be that in the first industrial revolution there was "myo-mechanization" and in the second, "neuro-mechanization." The first pierced barriers in human and animal myo-kinetic skills by replacing muscle power of horses and men; it did not replace human skill, preciseness, and above all thought. Automatic modes of production pierce the thought barrier, making man's mental skill and precision obsolescent in many new fields that heretofore were considered human activities.

Economic forces effect ever increasing degrees of obsolescence for man in industrial activities as scientists and engineers look upon any human being at work as a challenge to their ability to replace him by some automatic mechanical process. In the first industrial revolution man in his piecework labors became gradually separated from the whole product whereas now simple economics dictate his elimination entirely from hand assembly, record keeping, and practically everything else to which he cannot be entrusted because of his human frailties. Thus while providing numerous external improvements to his environment through discovery, mankind is faced with the expense of being subjugated to colossal domination by the philosophical, ethical, and social implications of discovery.

As Marxist and other philosophers have postulated, the mode in production of goods determines many of the social ethical criteria of a society. In viewing paths ahead for the healing art we must consider how current changes in mode of production will affect its tasks in the future. As both a science and art, medicine in its philosophy must share suspicion and distrust of present and future technology with the psychosociologists and those in humane letters. Medicine must school itself in the social or human effects of technology developing not only in society generally but within the profession. Technology within medicine already has produced an army of medical experts and specialists but has just about eliminated the general practitioner who will visit you at your home.

If medicine's future role lies beyond imminent partial or complete conquest of the external environmental, infectious, degenerative, and malignant diseases, it becomes allied to ekistic and ecologic forces affecting interiorization of man, where we must look to man's introspection as well as that which threatens him from his external environment. These forces in man, which will become the basis for paramount specialization in the healing art, are related to the choices man makes in progress through discovery. The choices are made at the expense of man's individuality, capacity for self-expression, and his ultimate aims; also involved are human biological egotism, interpersonal altruism, and need for gratitude accumulation among others and self-transcendence.

There has been no dramatic suddenness in man's transition to his automatic and defiled environment.* He did not retire one night to awaken to a new world. The transition occurred unsensed except by retrospective comparisons among those who knew well the old world. Until recently human beings spoke not of psychological and social implications of technology but of the marvels of science and technology. The shouts of those who recognized with suspicion the social portents of discovery were drowned by acclaims of the majority led to see St. George destroy the dragon of toil. Only time brought realization that the dragon may have been the hero.

The disappearance of large numbers of job classifications began gradually and gathered momentum through economics and appli-

*As a result, the fields of preventive medicine and public health have entered into a complex and somewhat strange world of environmental toxicology. Familiar concepts of cause and effect relationships (such as found in the infectious diseases) are changing. Among the infectious diseases there were recognizable symptoms, which could be related to exposure to a particular organism. In sharp contrast to this, toxic chemical and radiologic effects in the environment must be dealt with in terms of cumulative loss (often small such as in lead absorption from atmosphere) in relationship to chronic diseases or normal physiologic processes.

It is now well accepted among environmentalists that the recycling and in many instances reconversion of waste materials and energy to useful materials and purposes may be the only solution to defilement of air, water, and ground (conversion of sulphur oxides and hydrogen sulphide into fertilizers and flowers of sulphur; conversion of human waste into fertilizers and potable water; conversion of thermal pollution energy to some useful purpose).

170

cation of technology. This disappearance went unrecognized because of early retirements, national military commitments, shortened working hours, and an actual temporary increase in overall employment by creation of new industries. This first stage was followed by a static stabilization of total work force, which under control of government and labor extended demand for workers actually after their need had begun to decline.

Medical implications of the present static stage of industrial employment are few among the workers themselves except for minor changes in physiological and psychological functioning of individuals. These are due to lessened physical activity (hypokinetic effects), more impersonalized relationships at work, tensional or anxiety states due to centralization in a few individuals of responsibilities formerly shouldered by many, emotional insecurity in relationship to machines, and vacuums of communications among employees due to their lesser number and greater isolation or separation at work. Though minor in character these dysfunctions are mainly beyond the purview of the healing art either at the occupational health or community level since the conditions of work have been prestructured into the design and mechanism of modern work places. These pollutions of the emotional and physiological climate of the working man are not thought to have any serious sociological import. At present the adaptability of working human beings appears sufficient to counteract present work situations through more satisfying pursuits away from places of employment.

We must, however, look forward to medical implications of technological progress as this present static stabilized phase of human employment merges with the gathering momentum of man's self-made obsolescence, making him increasingly unemployable. It is within the context of this gathering momentum that a paramount specialty of *Interior* or *Interioristic Medicine* will be required in the healing art. This specialty dealing with man's introspection and self-transcendent needs may have its birth in what is now psychiatry but would gradually permeate the specialty of family practice and all branches of the healing art by virtue of its quantitative and universal need.

Today capability requirements for employment in intelligence, competence, and trainability are higher than the minimum of those days when papers were filed, ditches dug, and floors scrubbed—mostly by hand. Higher capability requirements already have placed large numbers of individuals in social categories considered *of* but not *in* our society. As scientists and engineers continue their work in industry the minimum capability requirements for employment rise. Thus additional members of society, willing but no longer capable, join the ranks of those *of* but not *in*. The logic of mathematics insists that only time becomes a factor before minimum capability requirements rise again, denying another segment of the population its social franchise, relegating them to some limbo of living with other obsolescent individuals. These will not be morons but persons of limited capability anxious to be useful and willing to work. Most will be heads of households and parents striving to guide their children to the best of their abilities. Their mental deficiency lies in inability to compete with industrial automatic processes and mentalities untrainable to fill a need in an automatic society. In the meantime the machinery that displaced them tirelessly continues to produce greater wealth and "comforts."

As previously indicated, the polity lacks practical means of reversing or overthrowing this type of "progress." Even with possession of such means there would be the impossible task of deciding which technical advances should be halted or which machines should be destroyed, since different members of society may wish destruction of different products of technological advancement. Thus we have reached the dilemma of no retreat or deviation on the present path of discovery; man must come to grips with where he is in the midst of discovery and its psychosociological implications.

We see in the not too distant future a picture of a fabulously wealthy society dominated by a colossus of almost unlimited production, its members receiving optimum benefits in medical maintenance of physiological integrity yet half or more of the populace unable to participate actively in its economics; people *of* but not *in* the society. Government's participation in making human beings economically useful through military service or works projects will be tested to ultimate capacity; also novel panaceic employment and retirement plans will be tried. In the midst of growing discontent and unhappiness government statistics may prove that the "dispossessed" have more automobiles, television equipment, and other wants than previous societies hoped or dreamed of. The enigma of unhappiness in the midst of plenty may even be translated as ingratitude among the dispossessed beneficiaries of an automated society's wealth.

Nowhere in history do we find successful responses in society to enforced leisure when large segments of its citizenry are economically useless. The citizens of Rome, freed from or denied labors of the fields converged on Rome to be fed and entertained by government in sports arenas. With slavery, the counterpart of automatic processes, Roman citizens lacked challenge, succumbed to uselessness, failed to grow as a society, and crumbled under the blow of barbarian invasions.

There are various alternatives in modern society that may be tried in overcoming the feeling of powerlessness; the malady of immensity, complexity, uncertainty; lack of transcendence among those dispossessed by a society geared to economic production. The creation of machinery had given hope for greater individuality among members of society; however gradually its members discovered a lessening of personal mastery over their lives, environments, and institutions. Cultural medications of the chemical variety and the shadows of television sets have provided only limited and temporary self-transcendence; in fact, these have deepened discontent, egocentricity, and introspection among members of a society suffering from economic "systemic" disease. Social medications in the form of shared fellowship among family, friends, relatives, and neighbors appear more difficult to obtain than in the days when means of travel and communication were less developed. Unlike in Roman times the cultural medication of crowds has been carefully structured on an economic scale so that the stadium and arenas become symbolic of construction, technology, and expansion as self-sufficient virtues.

Religious doctrines that served mankind with solace and as

anchors of truth and humility in storms of new discovery and social changes have been confounded by "accidental" details in discovery as they relate to the natural order, even though these new discoveries leave concepts and beliefs in the supernatural order basically unchanged (exploration of planets or discovery of nuclear energy do not contravert Genesis). There are those concerned with modern man's tensions, confusions, and loss of purpose who look for new sets of values in religion and ethics. Others feel there is nothing wrong with old religion and the values of love, equality, and human brotherhood of the past; they need only to be practiced in the Hebrew-Christian tradition. There are many caught in the social and existential crisis of the modern world who, dismayed by psychosocial results of science and technology, have lost credulity and power to affirm and believe in any ethical or religious values external to themselves or to their earthy, organic, natural, or animalistic existence. Individuals lacking vertical means of self-transcendence heretofore have sought horizontal means in the religion of work and reward; and to a lesser degree in the love bonds of communal relationships with family, friends, and relatives. When denied these horizontal relationships by a society becoming progressively automatic and complex, they become victims of a society suffering from multitude, complexity, and uncertainty.

In considering paths ahead for the art of healing we must postulate various modes of adaptation open to human beings in their adjustment (nongenetic) to psychosocial effects of progress in discovery and technology. The modes chosen will determine man's future characteristics, introspection, and the philosophy, tasks, or responsibilities of the healing art in its future contractural relationships with the polity. These future relationships may have less to do with man's physiological integrity or longevity than with providing man with depth and breadth to his existence, furnishing not only supportive therapy for living but cultural and philosophic acceptance of death.

We have mentioned solace in religiousness as one form of self-transcendence. We would add that although religion as an institution has often been subservient to dominant social, economic, and political forces it can supply as in the past the dynamics of protest against social evils of technological advancement. Religion had a very strong tradition of opposition to slavery from both biblical and post-biblical Judaism.* This tradition ameliorated the status of slaves at times when social, political, and economic conditions made abolition of slavery impossible. This means tradition could serve humanity in the *maladie* of technological slavery, black and white. Religion with belief in divinity and life hereafter becomes one of several courses open to human beings as a remedy for psychosocial disorder. Strong religious revivals conceivably could result from psychosocial effects of discovery and technology. These revivals have been connected with many crises in man's history. Christianity itself provided needed self-transcendence among Roman citizens and slaves during the fall of the empire.

Other courses open to humanity would be in the form of archaism; i.e., moratoriums on progress and return to practices in the distant past that seemed successful. Western civilization already has witnessed various attempts at archaism. In the eighteenth century Thoreau, alarmed by psychosocial evils of his time, speculated on the merits of return to the "natural life." Sects and cults of various sorts have advocated this approach in modern times.** In the midst of a modern technological economy spewing goods, "services," and "wealth," groups advocating back-to-nature are considered ludicrous, eccentric, unwashed, and more often crackpots. As mentioned earlier, the polity has no practical means for reversal, declaring a moratorium on "progress" and resulting

*Christianity, until the first quarter of the nineteenth century, was slow in recognizing forms of slavery (cultural, industrial, *et al.*) as a moral issue. From the time of the French Revolution, there had been a slow awakening in the world to its injustice. Christian sects, mainly Quakers and Protestants, set examples of Christian action against unjust human servitude. (Sailer, J. M. Handbuch der Christlichen Moral, II. Sämmtliche Werke, Sulzbach (1830-1941), XV, 196, 198). Canonical support, given slavery for centuries, raises the modern-day question of possible analogy between development of theological doctrine on slavery and doctrine relating to "anti-contraception." (Corpus Juris Canonici, Decreti Gratiani, Pars II, Causa XVII, Q. IV, Chapter 37. Proceedings of Second Vatican Council.

**The Dante G. Rossetti group in Victorian England also speculated on the practice and merits of the "natural life."

social or cultural changes. Even when catastrophe occurs, society does not reverse progress but rebuilds, seeking different routes of progress.

Another escape for humanity from its present technological bondage seems to lie in an upsurge of creativity with a renaissance in painting, literature, music, and philosophy—creation of new institutions of the art form. Human beings have retained creativity in the arts in spite of technical progress. While creativity has been associated with human adversity, in poverty and misery, societies as a whole have produced their finest creative works during periods of great social, economic, and political growth: at times when the societies' growth was able to support individual genius. Decadent periods in the arts have been associated with declining civilizations. Rome, during the Golden Age of Augustus, was in the early stages of decay, and little was produced in the way of artistic effort—most was a tired copy of an earlier Hellenic renaissance.

Upsurge in creativity as a form of transcendence is limited by the relatively few human beings who feel that their creative endeavors are sufficiently useful or worthwhile as a means of self-expression. Many individuals no matter how dedicated are unable to convince themselves or others, even their families, that their efforts in creative endeavor have value; many of these are content to view paintings or listen to music produced by a talented minority.*

Long-term hopes for solution of the problem have been based on belief in improvement of the species and education. Improvement through greater hominization no doubt will make man more

---

*Gustave Mahler's music has been described as a special kind of music for future generations. Perhaps Mahler anticipated by two centuries the need of an unhappy mankind for music in a parodic vein, as in his symphonic compositions the "Blumine" and "Todten Marsch" of *The Titan Symphony* and even in his *Kinder Todten Lieder.* These great works of a sometimes emotionally disturbed genius express great contrasts in thematic material, from Viennese hurdy-gurdy and military band music to musical expression of death and transfiguration. They would, to the author, seem suitable in furnishing many lost scales, triads, and chords in a nostalgic human existence. (For an exceptional commentary on the emotional matrix of Mahler's musical language, see Ernest Jones, *The Life and Works of Sigmund Freud.* New York: Basic Books, 1953.)

adaptable in relation to his scientific discovery and technology. While increase in educational opportunities will produce a better educated society it cannot soon produce a more intelligent one. Meanwhile the continual rise in the productive capability requirement for participation in an automated society makes many skills learned through training or education today obsolete tomorrow.

While man waits for his evolution to produce a higher capability factor, he must provide successful techniques in solving psychosocial problems that block fulfillment, without which man's life no matter how long becomes one of boredom and hopelessness. Human beings must have long-range goals. Religion, patriotism, tribes, families, and institutions have through the ages provided them, but we find many human beings today without any. Increasing numbers are denied individuality, self-expression; many find interpersonal altruism and even biological egotism difficult to express.

No one of the alternative modes of adaptation mentioned will be suitable to all people. There is already a large segment of our society that has either gradually withdrawn from or risen up in protest against the social complexities of overorganized social structures and ideologies based on compulsions and obsessions of industry, invention, and neat pious accountancy. Those who protest are less a challenge to or responsibility of the medical art than those who withdraw either into partial or total "neurotic deadness" or various stages of temporary self-transcendence through cultural (chemical) medications. Large numbers of persons today lack purpose and feeling of participation in goals beyond their daily existences; they also lack self-generating potentials. They have become victims of their own introspection. In giving up those real units of self, subject to isolation, hurt, and unhappiness, and accepting a neurotic bargain with modern society, these individuals epitomize the present malady of multitude, complexity, and uncertainty. Future efforts of the healing art directed toward humanistic care of patients must provide for a degree of specialism in human problems of interiorization resulting from broad social effects of science and technology.

So far, we have seen the response of the healing art to technological advance in priorities given to perfection of artificial organs, organ transplants, and the application of computer technology to aspects of diagnosis and delivery of medical care. These are open to serious question in light of the more compelling needs of a generally discontented, uncertain, unhappy society. These needs will become more pressing in proportion to the advances in science and technology, and the healing art cannot escape a large degree of responsibility placed by society on it and other professional groups for meeting these needs by a suitable philosophy in its educational system and medical research.

Technological advances within medicine and surgery continue and must be encouraged to ultimate useful and ethical applications. Since physicians like the rest of society can become subservient to invention, the question pertinent to medicine's future philosophy, education, and language is whether physicians should acquiesce entirely to technological subservience or through new invention free themselves for dedication to greater humanistic care of patients. Intimately bound to this is the problem of determining what shall be considered the highest skill of the future physician. Will it be comprised of or limited to technological, scientific engineering problems in management of difficult and esoteric problems in human physiological function? If so, will this be considered a higher skill than that required in total humanistic care of patients frequently delegated to para-medical persons or to those outside of the profession?* What ultimate purpose is served in maintaining the physiological integrity of a large number of patients who must on recovery return to a society that has made many already feel obsolete, unneeded as individuals?

If we judge by present circumstances in the healing art and by the voices of many in the polity, the highest skill in medicine still lies in the humanistic approach to patient care. It is this approach that offers hope, through future research, in giving the philosophy and language of medicine dynamic and useful principles in the optimum fulfillment of contractural relationships with the social order of man.

Discoursing on physicians in the art of healing, Plato advises

*Synanon, Alcoholics Anonymous, *et al.*

them that "there is no proportion or disproportion more productive of health and disease and of virtue and vice, than that between soul and body." The soul "convulses and fills with disorders the whole inner nature of man"; and when man is "eager in pursuit of learning, studying, teaching, disputing in private or public, disorders in the soul may dissolve the composite form of man and cause illness." Plato states further "we should not move the body without the soul or the soul without the body." We see in the discourse the holistic concept of man—one psychic whole, a single complete organic structure, and a social entity who seeks self-transcendence and ultimate aims by either religious, social, or other means.

We in medicine look upon the human being organically as a mechanism of great precision. In our attempts to maintain this precision we frequently forget the more delicate precision in the relationship between his organic housing and his membership in an evolving psychosocial order. Within this membership lie paths and tasks ahead for the healing art. It must harmonize (with *agape*) its tendencies and language with the behavioral or social sciences, with philosophy, religion, and all other disciplines concerned with man's place in the present or future "worlds" he discovers or invents. Only when man's hominization* has reached its ultimate can he walk with complete optimism, without jeopardy, in the direction of his invention and discovery. He then will have returned to Eden, enjoying existence without stress of disease or struggle with work and economic reward. In the meantime the healing art must provide him with supportive therapy for his chronic pessimism and discontent, much the same as good family physicians did prior to modern medicine's great technical advancements.

A British philosopher who four hundred years ago sought evidence in man's social evolution of development of a general therapeutic relatedness among human beings, stated simply his hopes

---

*Teilhard de Chardin, considered by many the great prophet of this century, believed that after man harnesses wind, wave, space, gravity and his own general environment, through hominization, he will harness love—then he will, again, have discovered fire.

and aspirations for his fellow man: "If every man would mend a man, then all of the world would be mended." The physician, over the centuries, on the whole has been concerned with and dedicated to the mending of bodies and minds. While there are modern practitioners who need to be reminded of holistic concepts in the practice of medicine, the great burden of the mending process in a torn, confused, and ravaged world obviously cannot be borne alone by the healing art; it must be shared, not only by those social sciences closely allied to medicine but by all sources of responsible professional leadership in society. This places moral responsibilities, spiritual and otherwise, upon educators, the clergy, lawyers, politicians, and businessmen.

CHAPTER VII

The American Character. Center for Study of Democratic Institutions. The Fund for the Republic, Inc. Santa Barbara, Calif., 1962.

American Friends Service Committee: *Who Shall Live? Man's Control over Birth and Death.* New York: Hill and Wang, 1970.

Bruhn, John G. "Human Ecology in Medicine." *Environmental Research,* Academic Press, New York and London, Vol. 3, No. 1 (January) 1970.

de Chardin, Teilhard, Pierre. Human Energy (trans.)Cohen, J. M. Ibid, de Chardin, Teilhard Pierre. Activation of Energy (trans.) Hague, René. New York: Harcourt, Brace, Jovanovich (1971).

Cole, Lamont C. "Man's Ecosystem." *Bio Science* (April) 1966.

Doxiadis, Constantinos A. *Ekistics: An Introduction to the Science of Human Settlements.* New York: Oxford University Press, 1968.

Doxiadis, Constantinos A. "Man and the Space Around Him." *Saturday Review* (Dec. 14), 1968.

Duhl, Leonard, J. "Health—20000 A.D." *American Journal Public Health* Vol. 59, No. 10, (Oct.) 1969.

Felton, J. S. "Individual Identity in a Continuing Industrial Revolution." *Archives of Environmental Health,* 14 (May), 1967.

Fitzgerald, James A. "Abortion on Demand." *Medical Opinion and Review* Vol. 6, No. 1, (January), 1970.

Goodwin, Richard N. "Reflections: Sources of the Public Unhappiness." *The New Yorker,* (   ), 1968, pp.

Henderson, J. J. and Mayo, Elton. "The Effects of Social Environment." *Journal of Industrial Hygiene,* Vol. 18, No. 7 (Sept.), 1936.

Hochuli, E. and Luongo, E. P. "Automation and the Obsolescence of Man." *Ind. Medicine and Surgery.* Chicago: Ind. Medicine Publishing Co. (Feb.), 1961.

Hoke, Lt. Cdr. Robert. "The Meaning of Work." *Archives of Environmental Health,* Vol. 16 (April), 1968.

Knight, James A. *Conscience and Guilt.* New York: Appleton-Century-Crofts, 1970.

Lindberg, D. A. B. *The Computer and Medical Care.* Springfield, Illinois: & Thomas, 1968.

Lindberg, D. A. B. *Computer Failures and Successes.* Birmingham: *Southern Medical Bulletin,* Vol. 57, No. 3, (Sept.), 1969.

The Republic of Plato (see Bibliography for Chap. I).

Toynbee, Arnold V. *A Study of History* (abridgement by D. C. Somerwell). London: Oxford University Press.

Wolman, Abel. "Water, Health and Society" in *Selected Papers by Abel Wolman.* Bloomington: Indiana University Press, 1969.

BIBLIOGRAPHY

General

Additional Reading

Philosophical Implications

Bergson, Henri. *Creative Evolution.* New York: Modern Library, Inc., 1944.

Copernicus, Nicolaus. *Three Copernican Treatises,* ed. Edward Rosen. New York: Dover Publications, Inc., 1959.

Darwin, Charles. *Origin of Species by Means of Natural Selection.* Garden City: Doubleday and Company, Inc., 1960.

Kant, Immanuel. *Critique of Practical Reason,* trans. Lewis W. Beck. New York: (Liberal Arts) Bobbs Merrill Company, 1956.

Mendel, Gregor. *Experiments in Plant Hybridization,* trans. The Royal Horticultural Society, London. Cambridge: Harvard University Press, 1925.

Newton, Isaac. *Sir Isaac Newton's Mathematical Principles of Natural Philosophy and his System of the World,* ed. Florian Cajori; trans. Andrew Motte, 2 vols. Berkeley: University of California Press, 1947.

Philosophers Speak for Themselves: Berkeley, Hume, and Kant. Chicago: University of Chicago Press, 1957.

Prosch, Harry. *Genesis of Twentieth Century Philosophy, The Evolution of Thought from Copernicus to the Present.* Garden City: Doubleday and Company, Inc., 1964.

Russell, Bertrand. *History of Western Philosophy.* New York: Simon and Schuster, Inc., 1959.

Dialectic Material

Marx, Karl. *Capital and Other Writings,* ed. Max Eastman. New York: Modern Library, Inc., 1932.

Pragmatist

James, William. *Essays in Pragmatism,* ed. Alburey Castell. New York: Hafner Publishing Company, 1957.

Pierce, Charles S. *Philosophical Writings of Pierce,* ed. Justus Buchler. New York: Dover Publications, Inc., 1965.

Analyst-Philosophers

Ayer, Alfred Jules. *Language, Truth, and Logic.* 2nd rev. ed. New York: Dover Publications, Inc., 1946.

Carnap, Rudolf. *Meaning and Necessity: A Study in Semantics and Modal Logic.* Chicago: University of Chicago Press, 1968.

Hare, R. M. *Language of Morals.* New York: Oxford University Press, 1952.

Russell, Bertrand. *Our Knowledge of the External World.* New York: New American Library, 1960.

Russell, Bertrand. *Mysticism and Logic.* Garden City: Doubleday and Company, Inc., 1957.

Existentialist

Beauvoir, Simone de. *The Ethics of Ambiguity,* trans. Bernard Frechtman. New York: Citadel Press, 1961.

Buber, Martin. *Between Man and Man,* trans. Ronald Gregor Smith, 2nd ed. New York: Charles Scribner's Sons, 1958.

Kierkegaard, Soren. *Fear and Trembling and Sickness Unto Death,* trans. Walter Lowrie. Garden City: Doubleday and Company, Inc., 1954.

Sartre, Jean Paul. *Existentialism,* trans. Bernard Frechtman. New York: Philosophical Library, Inc., 1947.

General Scientific

Einstein, Albert. *Out of My Later Years.* New York: Philosophical Library, Inc., 1956.

Psychiatric and General Scientific List

Alexander, F. (1943). "Fundamental Concepts of Psychosomatic Research: Psychogenesis, Conversion, Specificity." In, F. Alexander, T. M. French, *et al. Studies in Psychosomatic Medicine,* pp. 3-13. New York: Ronald Press, 1948.

Alexander, F. (1950). *Psychosomatic Medicine, Its Principles and Applications.* New York: W. W. Norton.

Allport, G. W. (1955). *Becoming. Basic Considerations for a Psychology of Personality.* New Haven: Yale University Press.

Ansbacher, H. L. and Ansbacher, R. R. (eds.) (1956). *The Individual Psychology of Alfred Adler. A Systematic Presentation in Selections from His Writings.* New York: Basic Books.

Bleuler, E. (1924). *A Textbook of Psychiatry.* Translated by A. A. Brill. New York: Macmillan, 1944.

Bowman, K. M., and Rose, M. (1954). "Do our medical colleagues know what to expect from psychotherapy?" *Am. J. Psychiat.,* 1:401.

Davis, K. (1938). "Mental Hygiene and the Class Structure." *Psychiatry,* 1:55.

Dewey, J. (1922). *Human Nature and Conduct. An Introduction to Social Psychology.* New York: Henry Holt.

Einstein, A. (1933). "On the Methods of Theoretical Physics." In, A. Einstein. *The World As I See It,* pp. 1-40. New York: Covici, Friede, 1934.

Einstein, A. (1941). "The Common Language of Science." In, A. Einstein. *Out of My Later Years,* pp. 111-113. New York: Philosophical Library, 1950.

Feigl, H. and Sellars, W. (eds.) (1949). *Readings in Philosophical Analysis.* New York: Appleton-Century-Crofts.

Ferenczi, S. (1913a). "The Symbolism of Bed-linen." In, S. Ferenczi. *Further Contributions to the Theory and Technique of Psycho-Analysis,* p. 359. London: Hogarth Press, 1950.

Frank, P. (1941). *Modern Science and Its Philosophy.* New York: George Braziller, 1955.

Freud, A. (1936). *The Ego and the Mechanisms of Defense.* New York: International Universities Press, 1946.

Freud, S. (1905a). "Fragment of an Analysis of a Case of Hysteria." In, *The Standard Edition of the Complete Psychological Worlds of Sigmund Freud.* Vol. VII, pp. 1-122. London: Hogarth Press, 1953.

Freud, S. (1910a). "Five Lectures on Psychoanalysis." In, *The Standard Edition of the Complete Psychological Works of Sigmund Freud.* Vol. XI, pp. 1-55. London: Hogarth Press, 1957.

Freud, S. (1910b). "The Antithetical Sense of Primal Words. A Review of a Pamphlet by Karl Abel, Uber den Gegensinn der Urworte (1884)." In, *Collected Papers.* Vol. IV, pp. 184-191. London: Hogarth Press, 1948.

Freud, S. (1914). "On the History of the Psychoanalytic Movement." In, *Collected Papers,* Vol. I, pp. 287-359. London: Hogarth Press, 1948.

Freud, S. (1915). "The Unconscious." In, *The Standard Edition of the Complete Psychological Works of Sigmund Freud.* Vol. XIV, pp. 159-204. London: Hogarth Press, 1957.

Freud, S. (1940). *An Outline of Psychoanalysis.* New York: W. W. Norton.

Fromm, E. (1951). *The Forgotten Language. An Introduction to the Understanding of Dreams, Fairy Tales and Myths.* New York: Rinehart.

Fromm, E. (1955). *The Sane Society.* New York: Rinehart.

Groddeck, G. (1927). *The Book of the Id Psychoanalytic Letters to a Friend.* London: C. W. Daniel, 1935.

Groddeck, G. (1934). *The World of Man, As Reflected in Art, in Words and in Disease.* London: C. W. Daniel.

Hardin, G. (1959). *Nature and Man's Fate.* New York: Rinehart.

Jackobson, R. (1957). "The Cardinal Dichotomy in Language." In, R. N. Anshen (ed.). *Language: An Enquiry into its Meaning and Function.* Chap. IX, pp. 155-173. New York: Harper.

Kemeny, J. G. (1959). *A Philosopher Looks at Science.* Princeton, Van Nostrand.

Kroeber, A. L. (1954). *Anthropology Today. An Encyclopedic Inventory.* Chicago: The University of Chicago Press.

Marx, K. (1944). "A Critique of the Hegelian Philosophy of Right." In, K. Marx. *Selected Essays*, pp. 11-39. Translated by H. J. Stenning. New York: International Publishers, 1926.

May, R. (1958). "The Origins and Significance of the Existential Movement in Psychology." In, R. May, E. Angel, and H. F. Ellenberger (eds). *Existence: A New Dimension in Psychiatry and Psychology*, Chapter I, pp. 3-36. New York: Basic Books.

Morris, C. W. (1946). *Signs, Language and Behavior*, New York: Prentice-Hall.

Morris, C. W. (1955). "Foundations of the Theory of Signs." In, O. Neurath, R. Carnap, and C. W. Morris (eds.). *International Encyclopedia of Unified Science*. Vol. I, pp. 77-137. Chicago: The University of Chicago Press.

Ogden, C. K., and Richards, I. A. (1930). *The Meaning of Meaning. A Study of the Influence of Language upon Thought and of the Science of Symbolism*. With Supplementary Essays by B. Malinowski and F. G. Crookshank. Third Revised Edition. New York: Harcourt, Brace.

Pirandello, L. (1919). "The Rules of the Game." Trans. Robert Rietty. In, *L. Pirandello: Three Plays*. Introduced and edited by E. Martin Browne. Harmondsworth, Middlesex: Penguin Books, 1959.

Rapoport, A. (1954). *Operational Philosophies Integrating Knowledge and Action*. New York: Harper.

Rogers, C. R. (1942). *Counseling and Psychotherapy, Newer Concepts in Practice*. Boston: Houghton Mifflin.

Rogers, C. R. (1951). *Client-Centered Therapy, Its Current Practice, Implications, and Theory*. Boston: Houghton Mifflin.

Roheim, G. (1943). *The Origin and Function of Culture*. Nervous and Mental Disease Monograph No. 69. New York: Nervous and Mental Disease Monographs.

Ruesch, J. (1959). "General Theory of Communication in Psychiatry." In, S. Arieti *et al.* (eds.) *American Handbook of Psychiatry*. Vol. I, Chapter 45, pp. 895-908. New York: Basic Books.

Ruesch, J., and Kees, W. (1956). *Nonverbal Communication*. Berkeley and Los Angeles: University of California Press.

Russell, B. (1948). *Human Knowledge, Its Scope and Limits*. New York: Simon and Schuster.

Sapir, E. (1921). *Language. An Introduction to the Study of Speech*. New York: Harcourt, Brace.

Schlick, M. (1935). "On the Relation Between Psychological and Physical Concepts," In, H. Feigl and W. Sellars (eds.). *Readings in Philosophical Analysis,* pp. 393-407. New York: Appleton-Century-Crofts, 1949.

Sellars, W. (1954). Some Reflections on Language Games. *Philosophy of Science*, 21:204.

Sigerist, H. E. (1951). "Primitive and Archaic Medicine." In, *A History of Medicine*. Vol. I. New York: Oxford University Press.

Sigerist, H. E. (1960). *Henry Sigerist on the Sociology of Medicine*. Edited by M. I. Roemer. Forword by J. M. Mackintosh. New York: MD Publications.

Spiegel, R. (1959). "Specific Problems of Communication in Psychiatric Conditions." In, S. Arieti *et al.* (eds.). *American Handbook of Psychiatry*. Vol. I, Chapter 46, pp. 909-949. New York: Basic Books.

Szasz, T. S. (1958). "Scientific Methods and Social Role in Medicine and Psychiatry." *A.M.A. Arch. Int. Med.*, 101:228.

Szasz, T. S., and Hollender, M. H. (1956). "A Contribution to the Philosophy of Medicine. The Basic Models of the Doctor-Patient Relationship." *A.M.A. Arch. Int. Med.*, 97:585.

Szasz, T. S., Knoff, W. F., and Hollender, M. H. (1958). "The Doctor-Patient Relationship in its Historical Context." *Am. J. Psychiat.*, 115:522.

Weiner, N. (1950). *The Human Use of Human Beings. Cybernetics and Society*. Garden City, N. Y.: Doubleday Anchor, 1954.

Weiner, N. (1960). "Some Moral and Technical Consequences of Automation." *Science*, 131:1355.

Wodger, J. H. (1952). *Biology and Language. An Introduction to the Methodology of the Biological Sciences Including Medicine*. Cambridge: Cambridge University Press.

Woodger, J. H. (1956). *Physics, Psychology and Medicine. A Methododological Essay*. Cambridge: Cambridge University Press.

Zilboorg, G. (1935). *The Medicine Man and the Witch During the Renaissance*. The Hideyo Nogushi Lectures. Baltimore: Johns Hopkins Press.

Zilboorg, G. (1941). *A History of Medical Psychology*. In collaboration with C. W. Henry. New York: W. W. Norton.

Zilboorg, G. (1943). *Mind, Medicine, and Man*. New York: Harcourt, Brace.

Public Health and Preventive Medicine

Blum, Henrik L. *Notes on Comprehensive Health Planning.* San Francisco, Calif.: Western Regional Office, American Public Health Association, 1967.

The Economics of Health and Medical Care. Ann Arbor: Bureau of Public Health Economics and Dept. of Economics, University of Michigan, 1964.

Fleming, D'Alonzo and Zapp. *Modern Occupational Medicine.* 1st ed. Philadelphia: Lea & Febiger, 1954.

Gafafer, W. M., D.S.C., Editor. *Occupational Diseases—A Guide to Their Recognition.* HEW-PHS-Supt. of Documents, U. S. Gov't. Printing Office.

Grant, Murray. *Handbook of Preventive Medicine.* 1st ed. Philadelphia: Lea and Febiger, 1967.

Hanlon, John. *Principles of Health Administration.* 5th ed. St. Louis: C. V. Mosby.

Leavell & Clark. *Preventive Medicine for the Doctor in His Community.* 2nd ed. New York: McGraw-Hill Book Co. Inc., The Blackstone Div. 1958.

Lilienfeld, Abraham M. and Alice J. Gifford, eds. *Chronic Diseases and Public Health.* Johns Hopkins Press, 1966.

Rosen. "History of Public Health." *M.D. Publications,* New York, 5:75.

Sartwell, Philip E. (ed.) *Preventive Medicine and Public Health.* 9th edition (formerly by Maxey and Rosenau). Appleton-Century-Crofts, 1965.

Sataloff, Joseph. *Hearing Loss.* Philadelphia: J. B. Lippincott Company, 1966.

Somera, Herman M., and Somers, Anne R. *Doctors, Patients and Care.* Washington, D.C.: The Brookings Institute, 1967.

Warshaw. *The Heart in Industry.* 1st ed., 1960, New York: Paul B. Hoeber, Inc., Medical Division of Harper & Bros.

Behavioral Sciences

Barnes, Elizabeth. *People in Hospitals.* London: Macmillan & Co., Ltd. (New York: St. Martin's Press, Inc.), 1961.

Becker, Geer, Hughes, and Strauss. *Boys in White.* University of Chicago Press, 1961.

Birren, James E. (ed.). *Handbook of Aging and the Individual: Psychological and Biological Aspects.* Chicago: University of Chicago Press, 1959.

Bloom, Samuel U. *The Doctor and His Patient: A Sociological Interpretation.* New York: Russell Sage Foundation, 1963.

188

Behavioral Sciences (continued)

Blum, Richard H., Sadusk, Joseph, and Waterson, Rollen. *The Management of Doctor-Patient Relationships.* New York: Blackstone Division, McGraw-Hill Book Company, Inc., 1960.

Brown, Esther Lucile. *New Dimensions of Patient Care.* New York: Russell Sage Foundation, 1964.

Cartwright, A. *Patients and Their Doctors: A Study of General Practice.* London: Rutledge and Kegan Paul, 1967.

Coser, Rose Laub. *Life in the Ward.* East Lansing: Michigan State University Press, 1962.

Duff, Raymond S., and Hollingshead, August B. *Sickness and Society.* New York: Harper & Row, 1968.

Feldman, Jacob J. *The Dissemination of Health Information.* Chicago: Aldine Publication Co., 1966

Folta, Jeannette R., and Deck, Edith S. (eds.). *A Sociological Framework for Patient Care.* New York: John Wiley and Sons, 1966.

Freeman, Howard E., Levine, Sal, and Reeder, Leo (eds.). *Handbook of Medical Sociology.* Englewood Cliffs: Prentice-Hall Inc., 1965.

Jaco, E. Gartly. *Patients, Physicians and Illness.* Free Press, Rev. ed., 1969.

Katz, Alfred H., and Felton, Jean Spencer (eds.). *Health and the Community.* The Free Press, 1965.

King, Stanley H. *Perceptions of Illness and Medical Practice.* New York: Russell Sage Foundation, 1962.

Mechanic, David. *Medical Sociology.* New York: The Free Press, 1968.

Minuchin, Salvador, *et al. Families of the Slums.* New York: Basic Books, 1967.

Paul, Benjamin. *Health, Culture and Community.* New York: Russell Sage Foundation, 1955.

Read, Margaret. *Culture, Health, and Disease.* London: Tavistock, 1966.

Scott, Richard W., and Volkart, Edmund H. (eds.). *Medical Care: Readings in the Sociology of Medical Institutions.* New York: John Wiley and Sons, 1966.

Sigerist, H. E. *On the Sociology of Medicine.* New York: M.D. Publications.

Skipper, James K., and Leonard, Robert C. (eds.). *Social Interaction and Patient Care.* Philadelphia: J. B. Lippincott Co., 1965.

Susser, M. W., and Watson, W. *Sociology in Medicine.* London: Oxford University Press, 1962.

SPECIALIZED (Health and Social Studies)
ADDITIONAL READING

Books

Duff, Raymond S., and Hallingshead, A. B. *Sickness and Society,* New York: Harper & Row, 1968.

Foster, George. *Traditional Cultures and The Impact of Technological Change.* New York: Harper & Row, 1962.

Harrington, Michael. *The Other American.* New York, Macmillan, 1962.

Lewis, Oscar. *La Vida.* New York: Random House, 1966.

Read, Margaret. *Culture, Health, and Diseases. Social and Cultural Influences on Health Programmes in Developing Countries.* Tavistock Publications: London, 1966.

Wirth, Louis. *The Ghetto.* University of Chicago Press: 1956.

Articles in Books

Cassel, John. "Social and Cultural Implications of Food and Food Habits," Chapter 16, p. 134-143.

Clark, Duncan W. and MacMahon, Brian (editors). *Preventive Medicine.* Boston: Little, Brown and Company, 1967.

Clark, Duncan W. "Social Welfare," Chapter 41, p. 781-812.

Cobb, Beatrex. "Why do People Detour to Quacks?" Chapter 30, p. 283-287.

Dubos, René. *Mirage of Health,* (Utopias, Progress, and Biological Change). (Paperback), Anchor Books. Parts I, II, VI, VII and VIII, 1961.

Jaco, E. Gartly (editor). *Patients, Physicians, and Illness.* Glencoe, Illinois, Free Press, 1958.

Klarman, Herbert E. "Financing Health and Medical Care," Chapter 40, p. 741-779.

Koos, Earl. "Metropolis—What City People Think of Their Medical Services," Chapter 13, p. 113-119.

Lederer, Henry. "How the Sick View Their World," Chapter 26, p. 247-256.

Marby, John. "Some Ecological Contributions to Epidemiology," Chapter 6, p. 49-54.

Mayer, Jean. "Nutritional Aspects of Preventive Medicine," Chapter 11, p. 187-207.

Parsons, Talcott, and Fox, Renee. "Illness, Therapy and the Modern Urban American Family," Chapter 25, p. 234-245.
Payne, Anthony M. M. "The Basis of Preventive Measures," Chapter 3, p. 19-38.
Stern, Bernhard J. "The Specialists and the General Practitioner," Chapter 36, p. 352-360.
Susser, M. W., and Watson, W. "Culture and Health," *Sociology in Medicine,* Oxford University Press, New York, 1962, p. 23.
White, Kerr L. "Patterns of Medical Practice," Chapter 43, p. 849-870.

Articles in Journals

American Journal of Public Health

Duhl, Leonard J. "Health Research and the University," Vol. 59, No. 1, 1969, p. 21-28.
Frank, Lawrence. "Interprofessional Communication," Vol. 51, No. 12, 1961, p. 1798-1804.
Harlon, John J. "An Ecological View of Public Health," Vol. 59, No. 1, 1969, p. 4-11.
Hinkle, Laurence E., Jr. "The Doctor, His Patient, and the Environment," Vol. 54, 1964, p. 11-17.
Kartman, Leo. "Human Ecology and Public Health," Vol. 57, No. 5, p. 737.
"Man-Made Environmental Hazards," Vol. 58, No. 11, 1968, p. 2043-59 (Parts I-III).

Archives of Environmental Health

Banta, James E. "Effecting Changes in Health Behavior in Developing Countries," Vol. 18 (February), 1969, p. 265-268.
Ingalls, Mary Tooke. "A Poverty Program Teacher Looks at Public Health," Vol. 16, 1968, p. 744-747.

Archives of General Psychiatry

von Mering, Otto, and Earley, L. William. "Major Changes in the Western Medical Environment," Vol. 13, 1965, p. 195-201.

Bull. New York Academy of Medicine

Bamberger, Lisbeth. "Health Care and Poverty" (December), 1966, p. 1140-1149.
White, Kerr L. "Personal Health Services: Defects, Dilemmas, and Directions" (April), 1968.

Ann. American Academy Political Social Science

Parsons, T. "Social Change and Medical Organization in the United States: A Sociological Perspective" (March), 1963, p. 21-23.

Atlantic Monthly

Drew, Elizabeth Brenner. "The Health Syndicate" (December), 1957.

GP

Ward, Donovan. "Meeting the Needs for Comprehensive Health Care" (July), 1965, p. 181-184.

Medical World News

Geiger, Jack. "Medicine Must Help Cure Ghetto's Ills" (May), 1968.
Gerber, Alex. "We Should Stop Expecting Doctors to Cure What Ails Society" (July 12), 1968.

Millbank Memorial Fund Quarterly

Brown, Howard J. "Delivery of Personal Health Services and Medical Services for the Poor—Concessions or Prerogatives," Vol. XLVI(1) (January), 1968, p. 203-225.
Elling, Ray H. "The Shifting Power Structure in Health," Vol. XLVI(1) (January), 1968, p. 119-143.

New England Journal of Medicine

Bergner, R., and Yerby, A. S. "Low Income and Barriers to the Use of Health Services," Vol. 278, 1968, p. 541-546.

Psychosomatic Medicine

Hinkle, L. E. "Ecological Observations of the Relation of Physical Illness, Mental Illness and the Social Environment," Vol. 23, 1961, p. 289-297.

Saturday Review

Michaelson, Michael G. "Medical Students: Healers Become Activists" (August 16), 1969, p. 41.

Scientific American

Lewis, Oscar. "The Culture of Poverty" (October), 1966.

World Medical Journal

Harlem, O. K. "Is it Necessary to Communicate With Patients?" Vol. 15, No. 4, 1968, p. 85-86.

Others

American Journal of Public Health
Annals of Medicine
APHA Legislative Newsletter
Archives of Environmental Health 1968-1969
Bookshelf on Social Sciences and Public Health—*APHA Journal* April 1959
    ,,   ,, the History and Philosophy of Public Health ,,   April 1960
    ,,   ,, Environmental Health ,,   April 1962
    ,,   ,, the Public Health Educator's Bookshelf ,,   April 1963
    ,,   ,, Maternal and Child Health ,,   April 1964
    ,,   ,, Mental Health ,,   April 1965
    ,,   ,, Dental Health ,,   April 1966
    ,,   ,, Reports of National Task Forces Project: Health Is a Community Affair ,,   April 1967
    ,,   ,, Foods and Nutrition ,,   April 1968
    ,,   ,, a Paperback Bookshelf in Public Health ,,   April 1968
    ,,   ,, Poverty and Health ,,   April 1969

British Journal of Social and Preventive Medicine
CERES (FAO Bulletin)
Current Bibliography of Epidemiology
Health Education Monographs
Health Service Research (Hosp. Res. and Ed'l Trust)
International Journal of Health Education
Journal of the American Medical Association
Journal of Chronic Diseases
Journal of Epidemiology
Journal of Health and Human Behavior
Journal of Occupational Medicine
Journal of School Health
Journal of Social Issues
Journal of Tropical Medicine and Hygiene
Journal of Tropical Pediatrics
Medical Care
Medical Care Review. School of Public Health, University of Michigan.
Medical Economics
Mental Health
Mental Health Digest
Millbank Memorial Fund Quarterly

National Communicable Disease Center's Weekly Report, *Morbidity and Mortality*, Dept. HEW/PHS, Atlanta, Ga.

Psychological Abstracts

Social Science and Medicine, Pergamon Press.

Sociological Abstracts

Trans-action

Washington Report. Weekly Legislative Newsletter

World Medical Journal

Miscellaneous Publications

Herzog, Elizabeth. *About the Poor—Some Facts and Some Fictions.* U. S. Department of Health, Education and Welfare, Children's Bureau Publication No. 451, 1967.

Lewis, Hylon. *Child-Rearing Among Low-Income Families.* Washington Center for Metropolitan Studies (June), 1961.

U. S. Commission on Civil Rights. *A Time to Listen—A Time to Act.*

Wolfgang, Marvine. *The Culture of Youth.* U. S. Department of Health, Education and Welfare, U. S. Government Printing Office, 1967.